Alternatives to Opioid Analgesia in Small Animal Anesthesia

Editors

CIARA BARR
GIACOMO GIANOTTI

VETERINARY CLINICS OF NORTH AMERICA: SMALL ANIMAL PRACTICE

www.vetsmall.theclinics.com

November 2019 • Volume 49 • Number 6

ELSEVIER

1600 John F. Kennedy Boulevard • Suite 1800 • Philadelphia, Pennsylvania, 19103-2899

http://www.vetsmall.theclinics.com

VETERINARY CLINICS OF NORTH AMERICA: SMALL ANIMAL PRACTICE Volume 49, Number 6

November 2019 ISSN 0195-5616, ISBN-13: 978-0-323-64141-8

Editor: Colleen Dietzler

Developmental Editor: Laura Kavanaugh

Veterinary Clinics of North America: Small Animal Practice (ISSN 0195-5616) is published bimonthly by Elsevier Inc., 360 Park Avenue South, New York, NY 10010-1710. Months of issue are January, March, May, July, September, and November. Business and Editorial Offices: 1600 John F. Kennedy Blvd., Ste. 1800, Philadelphia, PA 19103-2899. Customer Service Office: 3251 Riverport Lane, Maryland Heights, MO 63043. Periodicals postage paid at New York, NY and additional mailing offices. Subscription prices are $338.00 per year (domestic individuals), $662.00 per year (domestic institutions), $100.00 per year (domestic students/residents), $451.00 per year (Canadian individuals), $823.00 per year (Canadian institutions), $474.00 per year (international individuals), $823.00 per year (international institutions), and $220.00 per year (international and Canadian students/residents). To receive student/resident rate, orders must be accompanied by name of affiliated institution, date of term, and the *signature* of program/residency coordinator on institution letterhead. Orders will be billed at individual rate until proof of status is received. Foreign air speed delivery is included in all *Clinics* subscription prices. All prices are subject to change without notice. **POSTMASTER:** Send address changes to *Veterinary Clinics of North America: Small Animal Practice*, Elsevier Health Sciences Division, Subscription Customer Service, 3251 Riverport Lane, Maryland Heights, MO 63043. Customer Service (orders, claims, online, change of address): Elsevier Periodicals Customer Service, Elsevier Health Sciences Division **Subscription Customer Service 3251 Riverport Lane Maryland Heights, MO 63043. Tel: 1-800-654-2452 (U.S. and Canada); 314-447-8871 (outside U.S. and Canada). Fax: 314-447-8029. E-mail: journalscustomerservice-usa@elsevier.com (for print support); journalsonlinesupport-usa@elsevier.com (for online support).**

Reprints. For copies of 100 or more of articles in this publication, please contact the Commercial Reprints Department, Elsevier Inc., 360 Park Avenue South, New York, NY 10010-1710. Tel.: 212-633-3874; Fax: 212-633-3820; E-mail: reprints@elsevier.com.

Veterinary Clinics of North America: Small Animal Practice is also published in Japanese by Inter Zoo Publishing Co., Ltd., Aoyama Crystal-Bldg 5F, 3-5-12 Kitaaoyama, Minato-ku, Tokyo 107-0061, Japan.

Veterinary Clinics of North America: Small Animal Practice is covered in *Current Contents/Agriculture, Biology and Environmental Sciences, Science Citation Index, ASCA, MEDLINE/PubMed (Index Medicus), Excerpta Medica, and BIOSIS.*

Contributors

EDITORS

CIARA BARR, VMD
Diplomate, American College of Veterinary Anesthesia and Analgesia; Assistant Professor of Clinical Anesthesia, Department of Clinical Sciences and Advanced Medicine, School of Veterinary Medicine, University of Pennsylvania, Philadelphia, Pennsylvania, USA

GIACOMO GIANOTTI, DVM, DVSc
Diplomate, American College of Veterinary Anesthesia and Analgesia; Associate Professor of Clinical Anesthesia, Department of Clinical Sciences and Advanced Medicine, School of Veterinary Medicine, University of Pennsylvania, Philadelphia, Pennsylvania, USA

AUTHORS

MICHELE BARLETTA, DVM, MS, PhD
Diplomate, American College of Veterinary Anesthesia and Analgesia; Associate Professor, Department of Large Animal Medicine, College of Veterinary Medicine, University of Georgia, Athens, Georgia, USA

LUIS CAMPOY, LV CertVA, MRCVS
Diplomate of the European College of Veterinary Anaesthesia and Analgesia; Associate Clinical Professor, Chief of Anesthesiology and Pain Medicine, Department of Clinical Sciences, Cornell University, College of Veterinary Medicine, Ithaca, New York, USA

ANA C. CASTEJÓN-GONZÁLEZ, DVM, PhD
Diplomate, American Veterinary Dental College; Diplomate, European Veterinary Dental College; Department of Clinical Sciences and Advanced Medicine, School of Veterinary Medicine, University of Pennsylvania, Philadelphia, Pennsylvania, USA

HOPE DOUGLAS, VMD
Department of Clinical Sciences and Advanced Medicine, School of Veterinary Medicine, University of Pennsylvania, Philadelphia, Pennsylvania, USA

MOLLY J. FLAHERTY, DVM, CCRP
Department of Clinical Science, Ryan Veterinary Hospital of the University of Pennsylvania, Philadelphia, Pennsylvania, USA

MANUEL MARTIN-FLORES, DVM
Diplomate, American College of Veterinary Anesthesia and Analgesia; Associate Professor, Section of Anesthesiology and Pain Medicine, Department of Clinical Sciences, College of Veterinary Medicine, Cornell University, Ithaca, New York, USA

BEATRIZ MONTEIRO, DVM
PhD Candidate and Research Assistant, Department of Clinical Sciences, Faculty of Veterinary Medicine, Université de Montréal, Saint Hyacinthe, Quebec, Canada

PABLO E. OTERO, MV, PhD
Full Professor, Anesthesiology and Pain Management Department, Facultad de Ciencias Veterinarias, Universidad de Buenos Aires, Buenos Aires, Argentina

JAMES A. PERRY, DVM, PhD
Veterinary Cancer and Surgery Specialists, Milwaukie, Oregon, USA

DIEGO A. PORTELA, MV, PhD
Diplomate, American College of Veterinary Anesthesia and Analgesia; Assistant Professor, Anesthesiology and Pain Management, Department of Comparative, Diagnostic, and Population Medicine, College of Veterinary Medicine, University of Florida, Gainesville, Florida, USA

RACHEL REED, DVM
Diplomate, American College of Veterinary Anesthesia and Analgesia; Clinical Assistant Professor, Department of Large Animal Medicine, College of Veterinary Medicine, University of Georgia, Athens, Georgia, USA

ALEXANDER M. REITER, Dipl. Tzt., Dr med vet
Diplomate, American Veterinary Dental College; Diplomate, European Veterinary Dental College; Founding Fellow, AVDC Oral and Maxillofacial Surgery (OMFS), Full Professor of Dentistry and Oral Surgery, Chief of the Dentistry and Oral Surgery Service, Department of Clinical Sciences and Advanced Medicine, School of Veterinary Medicine, University of Pennsylvania, Philadelphia, Pennsylvania, USA

MARTA ROMANO, DVM, MSc, PhD
Diplomate, American College of Veterinary Anesthesia and Analgesia; Clinical Assistant Professor, Anesthesiology and Pain Management, Department of Comparative, Diagnostic, and Population Medicine, College of Veterinary Medicine, University of Florida, Gainesville, Florida, USA

HÉLÈNE L.M. RUEL, DMV, MSc
Diplomate of the American College of Veterinary Internal Medicine (Neurology); Department of Clinical Sciences, Faculty of Veterinary Medicine, Université de Montréal, Saint-Hyacinthe, Quebec, Canada

ALICIA M. SKELDING, DVM, MSc, DVSc
Diplomate, American College of Veterinary Anesthesiologists and Analgesia; Head of Anesthesiology, Toronto Animal Health Partners Emergency and Specialty Hospital, Toronto, Ontario, Canada

PAULO V. STEAGALL, MV, MS, PhD
Diplomate, American College of Veterinary Anesthesia and Analgesia; Associate Professor of Veterinary Anesthesia and Pain Management, Department of Clinical Sciences, Faculty of Veterinary Medicine, Université de Montréal, Saint Hyacinthe, Quebec, Canada

ALEXANDER VALVERDE, DVM, DVSc
Diplomate, American College of Veterinary Anesthesiologists and Analgesia; Associate Professor, Department of Clinical Studies, Ontario Veterinary College, University of Guelph, Guelph, Ontario, Canada

BONNIE D. WRIGHT, DVM
Diplomate, American College of Veterinary Anesthesia and Analgesia

Contents

Immunomodulatory Effects of Surgery, Pain, and Opioids in Cancer Patients — 981

James A. Perry and Hope Douglas

Surgery is the mainstay of therapy for canine and human solid cancers. Alarmingly, evidence suggests that the process of surgery may exacerbate metastasis and accelerate the kinetics of cancer progression. Understanding the mechanisms by which cancer progression is accelerated as a result of surgery may provide pharmacologic interventions. This review discusses surgery-induced cancer progression. It focuses on immunomodulatory properties of anesthesia and opioids and evidence that studies evaluating the role of opioids in tumor progression are indicated. It concludes by discussing why companion animals with spontaneously arising cancer are an ideal model for clinical trials to investigate this phenomenon.

Antiinflammatory Drugs — 993

Beatriz Monteiro and Paulo V. Steagall

This article reviews the mechanisms of action, clinical use, and recent scientific evidence for the use of nonsteroidal antiinflammatory drugs, grapiprant, acetaminophen (paracetamol), metamizole (dipyrone), and corticosteroids in pain management. The discussion is presented with an emphasis on the treatment of acute pain.

Alternatives to Opioid Analgesia in Small Animal Anesthesia: Alpha-2 Agonists — 1013

Alexander Valverde and Alicia M. Skelding

Alpha-2 agonists have potent analgesic effects, in addition to their sedative actions. Alpha-2 agonists provide analgesia through any of several routes of administration, including parenteral, oral, epidural or intrathecal and intraarticular, because of spinal and supraspinal actions. Systemic doses are short acting, whereas local administration at the site of action result in longer analgesic effects. The potent cardiovascular and respiratory effects of alpha-2 agonists should be considered when used as analgesics.

Acupuncture for the Treatment of Animal Pain — 1029

Bonnie D. Wright

Acupuncture is recognized to induce multifactorial changes in the neuro-regulatory aspects of pain physiology. Many aspects overlap with known receptor interactions of commonly used analgesic drugs, and acupuncture can increase the efficacy or replace the use of these pharmacologic pain treatments. This article discusses the currently recognized components of the pain pathways that are modified by acupuncture. It introduces the role of fibroblasts and fascia in mechanotransduction and discusses the ways in which this provides a link between the acupuncture needle and the nervous system and is a conduit for extracellular fluid movement, lymphatics, and the immune system.

Local anesthetics are the only class of drugs that can block transduction and transmission of nociception. Physical properties, mechanism of action, and pharmacokinetics of this class of drugs are reviewed in this article. The clinical use, such intravenous administration of lidocaine, and local and systemic toxic effects are covered. A review of current studies published in the human and veterinary literature on lidocaine patches (Lidoderm) and liposomal bupivacaine (Experal and Nocita) are discussed.

Adjuvant analgesics (ie, gabapentin, tramadol, and ketamine) are commonly used in small animal practice. Most of these drugs are prescribed for outpatients, when pain is refractory to classic analgesics (ie, local anesthetics, opioids, and nonsteroidal antiinflammatory drugs [NSAIDs]), or when contraindications exist to the administration of other analgesics, including NSAIDs. This article reviews the mechanisms of action, clinical use, potential adverse effects, and current evidence of adjuvant analgesics in the treatment of acute pain in companion animals. These drugs should be considered as alternatives aimed at reducing or replacing opioids.

Physical agent modalities can be effective in the perioperative period for controlling pain and inflammation. This article presents research-based evidence to support the use of these modalities in pain management and to reduce the use of pain medications, including opioids. The mechanism of action, applications, contraindications, and adverse effects of cryotherapy, pulsed electromagnetic field therapy, transcutaneous electrical nerve stimulation, and laser therapy are reviewed. Incorporation of 1 or more of these therapies in anesthesia pain management protocols can improve outcomes and reduce potential drug side effects.

VETERINARY CLINICS OF NORTH AMERICA: SMALL ANIMAL PRACTICE

FORTHCOMING ISSUES

January 2020
Minimally Invasive Fracture Repair
Karl C. Maritato and
Matthew D. Barnhart, *Editors*

March 2020
**Canine and Feline Respiratory Medicine:
An Update**
Lynelle Johnson, *Editor*

September 2020
**Feline Practice: Integrating Medicine and
Well-Being: Part II**
Margie Scherk, *Editor*

RECENT ISSUES

September 2019
Cancer in Companion Animals
Philip J. Bergman and Craig Clifford,
Editors

July 2019
Small Animal Infectious Disease
Annette L. Litster, *Editor*

May 2019
Advances in Palliative Medicine
Katherine Goldberg, *Editor*

SERIES OF RELATED INTEREST

Veterinary Clinics of North America: Exotic Animal Practice
https://www.vetexotic.theclinics.com/

THE CLINICS ARE NOW AVAILABLE ONLINE!
Access your subscription at:
www.theclinics.com

Erratum

An error was made in the July 2019 issue of *Veterinary Clinics: Small Animal Practice* (Volume 49, Issue 4, p. 703-718) in the article "Optimal Vector-borne Disease Screening in Dogs Using Both Serology-based and Polymerase Chain Reaction-based Diagnostic Panels" by Dr. Linda Kidd.

On page 713, under the subheading "serology" the sentence: "Serologic crossreactivity with spotted fever group Rickettsia also seems to occur in dogs infected with *Bartonella henselae*", with reference to reference number 78, is incorrect. They did not find evidence of serologic crossreactivity in that paper.

The print and online versions of the article have now been updated.

vetsmall.theclinics.com

Preface

From Crisis to Opportunity

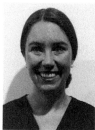 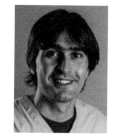

Ciara Barr, VMD   Giacomo Gianotti, DVM, DVSc
Editors

Currently, on average, 130 people die daily in the United States due to opioid over-dosage.[1] The opioid epidemic has become a national crisis due to the overprescribing of potent oral opioids in human medicine. To quote drug policy expert, Keith Humphreys[2]:

> The biggest misconception is that the US is normal in how it handles prescription opioids.

> So let's compare ourselves to another country. Japan, for example. Older population than us; you would think more aches and pains. Universal access to health care, so more opportunities to prescribe.

> So consider the amount of standard daily doses of opioids consumed in Japan. And then double it. And then double it again. And then double it again. And then double it again. And then double it a fifth time. That would make Japan No. 2 in the world, behind the United States.

> Every other developed country does at least as good or as poor a job as we do managing pain—while not using opioids at anywhere near the same level.

With the current opioid crisis raging, the pendulum has now swung from an abundance of opioids available to doctors to a shortage. The increased oversight regarding opioid prescriptions has affected not only hospital supplies but also veterinary access. Given this new restricted access and availability of opioids, we must expand our analgesic options in veterinary medicine. Furthermore, as increasing research is demonstrating, opioids may have negative impacts on immune function, gastrointestinal motility, and ultimately, patient outcomes with increased length of hospitalization in patients with high opioid consumption.

Vet Clin Small Anim 49 (2019) xi–xii
https://doi.org/10.1016/j.cvsm.2019.07.012
0195-5616/19/© 2019 Published by Elsevier Inc.

Both our increasingly limited access to opioids and growing knowledge of their detrimental effects require us to look beyond opioids for pain management in our patients. This issue of *Veterinary Clinics of North America: Small Animal Practice* presents cutting-edge research into the effects of opioids in surgical patients as well as a wide array of options for managing pain in order to reduce the use of opioids. We are grateful to our colleagues for their expertise in analgesic options to guide our treatment of patients as we navigate the opioid crisis and aim to reduce opioid use in the future.

Ciara Barr, VMD
Department of Clinical Sciences and
Advanced Medicine
University of Pennsylvania
School of Veterinary Medicine
Room 3005, 3900 Delancey Street
Philadelphia, PA, 19104, USA

Giacomo Gianotti, DVM, DVSc
Department of Clinical Sciences and
Advanced Medicine
University of Pennsylvania
School of Veterinary Medicine
Room 3007, 3900 Delancey Street
Philadelphia, PA, 19104, USA

E-mail addresses:
barr@upenn.edu (C. Barr)
gianotti@upenn.edu (G. Gianotti)

REFERENCES

1. Centers for Disease Control and Prevention. Opioid overdose: understanding the epidemic. Available at: https://www.cdc.gov/drugoverdose/epidemic/index.html. Accessed July 15, 2019.
2. Lopez G. America's huge problem with opioid prescribing, in one quote. Vox. September 18, 2017. Available at: https://www.vox.com/science-and-health/2017/9/18/16326816/opioid-epidemic-keith-humphreys. Accessed July 15, 2019.

Immunomodulatory Effects of Surgery, Pain, and Opioids in Cancer Patients

James A. Perry, DVM, PhD[a],*, Hope Douglas, VMD[b]

KEYWORDS

- Opioids • Cancer • Immunomodulation • Palliative care
- Perioperative immunosuppression

KEY POINTS

- Surgical removal of a primary tumor can accelerate metastatic progression at distant sites through a complex interaction between the primary tumor, its microenvironment, circulating tumor cells, the immune system, and sites of metastasis.
- Perioperative immunosuppression has been implicated as a key factor in surgery-associated accelerated tumor progression, and anesthetic/analgesic protocol may influence, in part, this phenomenon.
- Opioid drugs, specifically strong μ-agonists, have immunomodulatory properties that have been shown to inhibit natural killer cell function, alter macrophage phenotype, and reduce cell-mediated immunity.
- Multimodal anesthetic and analgesic protocols designed to reduce the requirement of opioids in the perioperative setting may improve cancer outcomes. Clinical trials to assess such protocols are under way, with more needed.

INTRODUCTION

Management of pain in cancer patients, whether in the perioperative setting for cancer surgery or for long-term management of chronic cancer pain in the palliative setting, is an integral component of clinical oncology (**Fig. 1**). The management of oncologic pain is an evolving practice as understanding of the interaction of pain and its treatment with the immune system, disease progression, and clinical outcomes in cancer patients improves.

In simple terms, *pain*, as defined by the Association for the Study of Pain, is "an unpleasant sensory and emotional experience that is associated with actual or potential

The authors have no conflicts of interest to report.
[a] Veterinary Cancer and Surgery Specialists, 10400 Southeast Main Street, Milwaukie, OR 97222, USA; [b] University of Pennsylvania, Department of Clinical Sciences and Advanced Medicine, School of Veterinary Medicine, 3900 Delancey Street, Philadelphia, PA 19104, USA
* Corresponding author.
E-mail address: drperry@vcsspdx.com

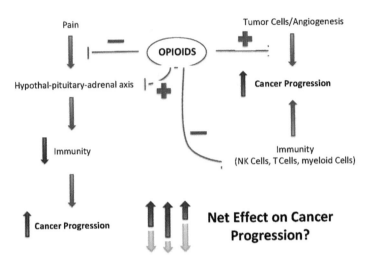

Fig. 1. Schematic interplay that opioids may have on the immune system and cancer progression. Studies suggest that the dominant immunosuppressive force is uncontrolled pain. When pain is managed using opioids, however, there may be confounding immunosuppressive properties of opioids themselves, leading to accelerated cancer progression, albeit likely less than that if pain was left uncontrolled. A balance may come with use of other nonimmunosuppressive analgesia methods, such as effective locoregional anethesthetics, NSAIDs, and/or non–μ-opioid receptor agonists, such as buprenorphine. (*Adapted from* Boland, J.W. & Pockley, A.G. Influence of opioids on immune function in patients with cancer pain: from bench to bedside. *British journal of pharmacology* 175, 2726-2736 (2018); with permission.)

tissue damage." Both physical (nociceptive) and emotional aspects of pain are intertwined within the immune system and can have variable effects on outcomes in cancer patients.

The immune system has a crucial role in cancer surveillance and limiting tumor progression within an established primary tumor and its associated metastases. This has been demonstrated both experimentally and in clinical patients where stimulation of the immune system can result in improved survival, whereas inhibition of the immune system can have detrimental effects on outcomes.

Pain itself is immunosuppressive. This occurs through activation of the hypothalamic-pituitary-adrenal axis leading to secretion of immunosuppressive catecholamines, corticosteroids, and other humoral factors. Blocking pain via local anesthetics, anti-inflammatory agents, and opioids can abrogate this immunosuppressive cascade. Certain analgesics however, while blocking pain-induced immunosuppression through their direct analgesic properties, can have immunomodulatory properties in their own right. Opioids, are one such class of drug.

The purpose of this review is to focus on the physical aspects of pain (nociception) in the perioperative period of cancer treatment and on how pain and its management may influence outcomes. How surgical injury and primary tumor removal can influence cancer outcome (so-called surgery-induced cancer acceleration or postsurgery metastatic acceleration) is discussed first; then, anesthesia and the role opioids may play in this process are focused on. Much of the data presented have been obtained from in vitro work, laboratory animal models, and human retrospective studies. Veterinary studies currently are being performed, however, to verify and expand these findings in companion animals and to model this phenomenon further for translation to human oncology.

SURGERY ACCELERATES PROGRESSION OF METASTATIC DISEASE

The hypothesis that cancer surgery accelerates tumor progression elsewhere in the body dates back to the turn of the twentieth century.[1] Experimental evidence support-ing this clinical observation soon followed using transplantable mouse tumor models. One such study, published in 1913, found that mice undergoing incomplete surgical removal of an inoculated tumor had a larger metastatic disease burden compared with nonoperated control mice.[2] In these early experiments, sham surgeries were not performed; therefore, differentiating the impact of the surgical process itself versus removal of the primary tumor (ie, concomitant tumor resistance[a])[3] for the observed re-sults was not possible. Since these early observations and experimental studies, remarkable progress, albeit incomplete, has been made to understand the underlying mechanisms involved in surgery-accelerated tumor progression. As would be ex-pected, the process of surgery-accelerated tumor progression is highly complex and multifactorial. Conceptually, the process of surgery-accelerated tumor progres-sion can be compartmentalized into immunologic and nonimmunologic processes, both of which can be influenced by intrinsic and extrinsic factors to the primary tumor and its microenviroment.

First, in a process termed, *concomitant tumor resistance*, the presence of the pri-mary tumor itself may inhibit the progression or even development of metastatic foci through several mechanisms. The most well-documented mechanisms of concomitant tumor resistance include (1) immunomodulation by the primary tumor and its microenvironment, (2) shifts in proangiogenic vs antiangiogenic states both locally and at distant sites, and (3) sequestration of protumor nutrients by the primary tumor from potential or early metastatic foci, or so-called atrepsis theory[b]. This dis-cussion is focused on modulation of the immune system and angiogenesis because these are points where anesthesia and opioids may influence tumor control and pro-gression. The focus is also shifted from the competition/atrepsis theory due to recent studies rebuking this mechanism of concomitant tumor resistance.[4]

Although immunomodulation is currently an area of intense interest in cancer biology and therapy and is likely an important factor in concomitant tumor resistance and surgery-induced cancer acceleration, studies in immunocompromised mice have proved that concomitant tumor resistance and surgery-induced cancer acceleration occurs, at least in part, irrespective of the immune system. In this setting, alterations in angiogenesis seem to primarily explain the mechanistic landscape. Numerous studies have shown that primary tumors secrete or induce the secretion of both proan-giogenic and antiangiogenic factors. The concentrations of proangiogenic and antian-giogenic factors often differ within the primary tumor relative to distant sites, and removal of a primary tumor can shift the systemic angiogenic balance from one that is antiangiogenic to proangiogenic. This was recently shown experimentally using an immunocompromised mouse model of osteosarcoma where removal of the

---

[a] Concomitant tumor resistance is a phenomenon characterized by resistance within a host to the development and/or progression of secondary implantable tumors in cases of experimental models or metastasis in the clinical setting. Mechanisms of concomitant tumor resistance are both immuno-logic and nonimmunologic in nature.

[b] Atrepsis theory is based on the theory that a primary tumor is a trap for glucose, nitrogen, and other essential nutrients, thereby starving or outcompeting early metastasis for resources.

primary tumor resulted in the reduction of endostatin (an antiangiogenic protein) concentrations with significant promotion of angiogenesis and increases in pulmonary metastatic foci.[5,6] Importantly, the prometastasis effects of removing the primary tumor in that study were abrogated with perioperative treatment with an endostatin analogue.[5]

A shift in proangiogenic versus antiangiogenic balance has also been observed in studies involving immunocompetent subjects. Specifically, in a study comparing concentrations of a proangiogenic compound, vascular endothelial growth factor (VEGF) in human patients undergoing surgery for gastric cancer, VEGF concentrations were significantly elevated after surgery.[7] This increase in VEGF concentration was exacerbated in patients undergoing open abdominal surgery compared with minimally invasive methods.[8] This latter study suggests a means for limiting the effects of tumor surgery on VEGF concentration increases, and a further understanding of how less invasive surgeries limit VEGF production is a current topic being actively investigated in both human and preclinical studies.

The effect of surgical invasiveness has been shown not only to alter VEGF concentrations but also to influence long-term outcomes in patients undergoing surgery. In a separate study comparing open versus laparoscopic resection of colonic adenocarcinoma, an overall improvement in cancer-free survival was observed in patients who underwent minimally invasive surgical procedures compared with open surgical treatments.[9] Whether the benefit in cancer-free survival in these studies is a direct result of reduction in proangiogenic factors versus other mechanisms, including immunomodulation, remains to be determined.

Another mechanism by which surgery may cause cancer acceleration, or with less invasive surgical procedures limit the degree of surgery-induced cancer acceleration and perceived concomitant tumor resistance, is via modulation of the immune system. Specifically, surgical trauma seems to induce local and systemic inflammatory responses, leading to immunosuppression and potential tumor escape from immune surveillance. In an elegant study evaluating spontaneous pulmonary metastasis in immunocompetent mice with syngeneic B16 flank melanoma, Da Costa and colleagues[10] showed that removal of the primary tumor exacerbated metastasis, and the addition of either a laparotomy or simulated laparoscopy (CO_2 peritoneal insufflation for 20 minutes) further potentiated the effect of primary tumor removal. This study also showed that open laparotomy had a greater prometastatic effect than simulated laparoscopy, further supporting the finding of the previously mentioned study by Lacy and colleagues[9] comparing open versus laparoscopic colonic adenocarcinoma removal in people. Da Costa's group went further to show that removal of the primary tumor led to the expansion of immunomodulatory macrophages within the spleen and diminished natural killer (NK) cell function, and these immune changes were exaggerated when simulated laparoscopy and, to a larger extent, laparotomy were performed. All mice in these studies received similar anesthesia (halothane) without additional analgesia.

Although these studies have set the stage to show that concomitant tumor resistance and postsurgery metastasis acceleration do occur and that both immunomodulation and alterations in angiogenesis play a role in these phenomena, they were not designed to determine whether manipulations in anesthetic or analgesic protocols could alter these observations.

In the subsequent sections, we specifically discuss how anesthesia and analgesia protocols may influence cancer outcomes with a focus on opioids. Evidence suggest that despite their ability to mitigate pain, opioids also have direct effects on cancer and immune cells that may promote tumor/metastasis progression.

ANESTHETIC PROTOCOL INFLUENCES PROGRESSION-FREE SURVIVAL—A ROLE FOR OPIOIDS?

In people, and likely similarly in dogs, approximately 80% of patients undergo some form of anesthesia, whether for diagnostic or treatment purposes, during the course of their cancer treatment of solid tumors. Accumulating evidence suggests alterations in the immune system as a result of anesthesia contribute to cancer progression. Several studies, most retrospective in nature, have shown also that the degree at which these alterations effect cancer progression can be related to specific anesthesia protocols utilized. Differences in outcomes have been observed when comparing type of anesthetic agent used (ie, inhalational vs total intravenous [IV] anesthesia), methods of analgesia administration (ie, IV opioid analgesia vs epidural analgesia) and whether additional drugs or treatments, such as allogeneic blood products, nonsteroidal anti-inflammatory drugs (NSAIDS), and β-blockers, were utilized.[11]

In a large retrospective study comparing total IV anesthesia to volatile inhalational anesthesia, controlling for known confounders in patients receiving elective cancer surgery, researchers found that mortality was approximately 50% greater in patients receiving inhalant anesthesia versus total IV anesthesia with an adjusted hazard ratio of 1.46.[12] Patients in the total IV anesthesia group received continuous infusions of propofol and remifentanil throughout the surgical procedure whereas patients in the inhalant anesthesia group received sevoflurane or isoflurane and supplementary opioids at the discretion of the anesthetist. Because both groups received some form of opioid, comparisons between opioid-containing and completely opioid-free protocols could not be made. Additionally, descriptions of the specific types and dosages of opioids used in the inhalant anesthesia group were not reported. Therefore, it is unclear whether opioids use may have confounded the results that showed a survival advantage for patients receiving total IV anesthesia over those receiving inhalant-based anesthesia.

Similarly, in a study comparing outcomes in human patients with cutaneous malignant melanoma undergoing surgical excision with local versus general anesthesia, the type of anesthesia performed was found to be an independent prognostic factor—patients undergoing local anesthesia in the absence of inhalant anesthetics showed improved survival compared with their general anesthesia control cohort.[13] Similar to the study discussed previously by Wigmore and colleagues,[12] opioid use was not compared between groups or analyzed as a confounding variable.

The role for locoregional anesthesia was also explored by Exadaktylos and colleagues[14] in a retrospective study investigating whether the choice of anesthetic technique could affect the outcome of breast cancer patients. In this analysis, patients undergoing mastectomy and axillary clearance for breast cancer received either paravertebral block and general anesthesia followed by paravertebral infusion for 48 hours or general anesthesia alone followed by postoperative patient-controlled analgesia with morphine. The investigators found that the use of the paravertebral block for breast cancer surgery reduced the risk of recurrence or metastasis 4-fold during a 2.5-year to 4-year follow-up period. Furthermore, in a retrospective study by Hiller and colleagues,[15] patients receiving an effective epidural for postoperative pain management after gastric and/or esophageal cancer surgery had a statistically improved 2-year survival rate compared with patients receiving IV opioid analgesia and no epidural. In the same study, the 2-year survival rate was also found to be specifically decreased in patients receiving allogeneic blood transfusions, which have also been implicated in immunosuppression and potential cancer acceleration.[15,16] It cannot be deduced from the available data in the Hiller and colleagues study whether the survival advantage in the epidural group was the result of improved pain management overall or whether the addition of IV opioid analgesia in the nonepidural group had the dominant effect.

In vivo animal studies aimed at determining the mechanism behind such effects of clinical anesthetic protocols on cancer outcomes observed in clinical studies suggest that exposure to volatile anesthesia leads to immunosuppression. Animal studies evaluating the immunomodulatory effects of inhalant anesthetics have shown suppression NK cell activity, reduced recruitment of macrophages and dendritic cells, and decreased helper T-cell activity.[11] Although a majority of these studies were performed in either mice or rats, one such study was performed in dogs, which confirmed a decreased NK cell function during isoflurane-based anesthesia in an outbred immunocompetent animal model.[17] To the authors' knowledge, and as stated by Dubowitz and colleagues,[11] no such clinical studies have specifically related the impact of inhalant anesthetics used during cancer surgery on immune function to cancer outcome.

As discussed in more detail later, similar to inhalant anesthetics, opioids have also been found to have immunosuppressive functions in vitro. Therefore, opioids may potentiate the effects of volatile anesthetic agents but in vivo studies looking specifically at opioid-free anesthetic protocols while controlling for all other variables, to the authors' knowledge, have yet to be performed. Until randomized prospective studies have been performed, the ultimate clinical effect remains speculative.

SPECIFIC IMMUNOMODULATORY AND POTENTIALLY CANCER-PROMOTING EFFECTS OF OPIOIDS

Opioids are among the most effective and powerful analgesics available for treating pain. Opioids exert their canonical analgesic effects via binding to opioid receptors in the central nervous system. Opioid receptors are located throughout the body, however, which contributes to the numerous nonanalgesic effects of opioid administration. Of particular interest to cancer biology and tumor microenvironment, opioids interact with the endothelium, tumor cells, and inflammatory cells via opioid receptor and non-opioid receptor mediated mechanisms.[18]

As such, opioids have both direct and indirect effects on the immune system and inflammation. Opioids, often acting through the μ-opioid receptor expressed on immune cells (granulocytes, monocytes/macrophages, lymphocytes, and NK cells),[19] have been shown to have a negative impact immune function, increase the risk for infection, and reduce overall survival times in numerous rodent models of cancer.[20,21] Initial evidence to suggest opioids induce immunosuppression came through studies showing increased susceptibility to infection in individuals using or abusing opioids.[22] Such correlations have been observed in several more recent retrospective studies looking at morphine and other μ-agonist use and risk of infections. In a retrospective study looking at chronic μ-opioid use (morphine, oxycodone, or fentanyl), as measured in oral morphine equivalent daily dose, a 2% increase in risk of infection for every 10-mg rise in equivalent dose was observed.[23]

Proposed mechanisms of opioid-induced immunosuppression include indirect suppression through the modulation of the hypothalamic-pituitary-adrenal axis via μ-opioid receptors within the central nervous system and direct inhibition of immune cell function within both the innate and adaptive immune systems.[c] The net effect of these mechanisms includes a reduction in circulating immune cell numbers, suppression of NK cell cytotoxicity, decreases in phagocytic and respiratory burst activity of innate immune cells, impaired immunocyte migration and chemotaxis, and a shift toward anti-inflammatory cytokine profile in response to immune stimulation.

Within the central nervous system, the acute immunosuppressive effects of morphine have been shown to occur through 2 principal pathways. The first is induction of the release of immunosuppressive biological amines through the sympathetic nervous system by acting on the periaqueductal gray matter[24] and the second is activation of dopamine D1 receptors in the nucleus accumbens shell, resulting in the release of neuropeptide Y and a reduction of NK cell cytotoxicity.[25,26] Chronic exposure of the central nervous system to morphine also activates the hypothalamic-pituitary-adrenal axis, much in the same way pain itself can induce immunosuppression.[27] Activation of these centrally acting pathways leads to different means of immunosuppression. Specifically, as shown through a series of experiments by Fecho and colleagues,[24] acute morphine administration in rats induced adrenal cortex–dependent suppression of peripheral blood lymphocyte activation and sympathetic nervous system/β-adrenergic–dependent suppression of splenic lymphocytes, whereas inhibition of splenic NK cell cytotoxicity occurred independent of both the sympathetic nervous system and adrenal cortical function.

As discussed previously and further suggested by observations in NK cells by Fecho and colleagues, opioids can interact independent of the central nervous system and directly with cells of the immune system. In addition to NK cell function, the cell types most implicated in direct opioid-mediated immunosuppressive effects include antigen-presenting cells (ie, dendritic cells), macrophages, and T cells. Such effects can be mediated directly though μ-opioid receptors expressed on the immune cells or through naturally occurring immunoreceptors, such as Toll-like receptors. Additionally, μ-opioid and other immunoreceptor expression on immune cells is not fixed and can be up-regulated by inflammatory cytokines, including tumor necrosis factor (TNF)-α, interleukin (IL)-1, and IL-6 (ie, cytokines that are increased in serum secondary to surgical trauma).[28,29] Specifically, the acute-phase cytokine TNF-α has been shown to up-regulate μ-opioid receptor expression in primary human T cells, polymorphonuclear cells, and dendritic cells.[29] Together, these studies suggest that that not only can opioids act on immune cells but also surgical trauma–associated proinflammatory cytokine release may potentiate the effect of opioids on immune cells.

Opioid use in laboratory animal models of cancer can lead to accelerated tumor progression not to mention several retrospective clinical studies in human patients have shown a negative impact on cancer outcomes of opioids in the treatment of perioperative surgical pain and for the treatment of chronic cancer pain,[14,30–32] and certain μ-opioid receptor polymorphisms have been linked to differences in outcomes in human breast cancer patients.[33] Additionally, in a recent study evaluating the use of low-dose naltrexone, a pure opioid antagonist, as an adjuvant to carboplatin chemotherapy in dogs with malignant mammary carcinoma therapy, an improved cancer-free survival was observed.[34]

---

[c] The innate immune system consists of epithelial barriers, including the gut and its microbiome, phagocytes, dendritic cells and NK cells. The adaptive immune system is predominated by B cells and T cells, which, importantly, are tightly regulated by itself the innate immune system.

Mechanistically, opioids also have been shown to promote angiogenesis and directly promote tumor growth and metastasis in a μ-opioid receptor–dependent fashion.[32,35] Gupta and colleagues[32] found that morphine, like VEGF, promotes angiogenesis by stimulating endothelial cell proliferation through the mitogen-activated protein kinase/extracellular signal–regulated kinase signaling pathway. In addition, the researchers found that morphine inhibited apoptosis and encouraged cell-cycle progression in endothelial cells.[36]

Opioids also can exert effects through direct binding to opioid receptors on neoplastic cells. Opioid receptors have been found on tumor cells from glioma and carcinomas, such as colon, breast, lung, pancreatic, thyroid, and endometrial cancers.[19] Mathew and colleagues[20] found a 5-fold to-10-fold increase in μ-opioid receptor expression in lung tissue from patients who had non–small cell lung carcinoma. Singleton and Moss[31] found that the expression of μ-opioid receptor in human lung cancer is significantly increased relative to adjacent control tissue and is approximately 2-fold higher in cases of metastatic lung cancer relative to that in individuals with nonmetastatic cancer.[19] In the Mathew and colleagues[20] study, morphine increased the in vitro growth of Lewis lung carcinoma, and cancer growth was inhibited by silencing the μ-opioid receptor expression or by administration of methylnaltrexone (a μ-opioid receptor antagonist).

The type of opioid administered can cause different effects on the immune system. In a study by Franchi and colleagues,[37] the immune effects of buprenorphine, a partial κ/μ-agonist, was compared with fentanyl and morphine in a rat model of surgical stress. Buprenorphine was able to prevent the neuroendocrine and immune system effects (particularly inhibition of NK cell activity) and reduce the degree of tumor metastasis observed by the surgical stress and morphine administration. Additionally, the chemical structure of the opioid may play a role in the level of immune suppression. Although morphine has been shown to be immunosuppressive, another μ-agonist, hydromorphone, does not seem to have this property due to a substitution of a carbonyl group at C-6.[38] Common to a majority of studies, regardless of mechanism, is that morphine and some other strong μ-agonist opioids (including endogenous opioids) are immunosuppressive and potentially promote metastasis. Importantly, not only can the type of opioid be a factor influencing nonanalgesic effects but also the route, dose, and duration of opioid administration likely play a role.

Despite the growing body of evidence suggesting the immunosuppressive role of opioids and their potential to contribute to tumor metastasis, there has been some contradictory evidence. Doornebal and colleagues[39] used a murine model for metastatic breast cancer and found that the analgesic dose of morphine did not affect tumor growth, the immune cell composition within the tumor, angiogenesis, or metastasis in mice undergoing mastectomy. This study highlights the inconsistencies in opioid administration between studies with regard to dosage, route of administration, and duration of administration. Additionally, it is important to keep in mind when extrapolating between murine and human studies that morphine metabolism varies between rodents and humans. In rodents, the main metabolite of morphine is inactive morphine-3-glucoronide compared with morphine-6-glucoronide in people, which is highly analgesic.[40] Although canine morphine metabolism is believed to be similar to that of humans, morphine-6-glucoronide was not detected in canine plasma during a pharmacokinetic evaluation of morphine in dogs.[41,42] These conflicting results further support the need for additional experimental and clinical studies to explore the perioperative use of opioids and the impact on immune function and tumor metastasis in veterinary and human patients.

SUMMARY

Surgery, anesthesia, nociception, and opioid use alone or in combination cannot solely explain the phenomenon of postsurgery metastasis acceleration, and it cannot be over-emphasized that these processes are multifactorial and incompletely understood. As such, strong recommendations as to how clinicians should treat patients based on currently available evidence is not possible. Ultimately, clinicians should implement treatment decisions based on individual risk-benefit analyses and adjust standard protocols as more evidence-based recommendations become available. It is likely that uncontrolled pain-induced immunosuppression is more detrimental to a patient's immune system and outcomes than the effect of opioid induced immunosuppression in a setting where pain is well managed. Therefore, pain management is of utmost importance. Based on the available evidence, however, reducing or replacing the need for opioids, through the implementation of less invasive procedures when possible and through the use of locoregional analgesia and other pharmacologic agents with potentially less off-target detrimental effects on the body's immune and other systems, could be strived for. Although opioid-free anesthesia is not likely to be a silver bullet when it comes to cancer surgery, it may be the start to understanding how improvements in cancer outcomes can be made.

Because controlled prospective studies evaluating the effects of anesthesia protocol on cancer outcomes in people are difficult, based on cost, patient longevity after cancer surgery, and emotional aspects of pain and opioid use, the utilization of veterinary patients with spontaneous cancers in well-controlled clinical trials may help provide an answer to these important questions. The goal of such trials will be not only to determine if opioid-free cancer surgery can improve survival in veterinary cancer patients but also to evaluate on a mechanistic basis looking at immune function at the cellular level in an outbred population of animals with cancer.

REFERENCES

1. Halsted WSI. The results of radical operations for the cure of carcinoma of the breast. Ann Surg 1907;46:1–19.
2. Tyzzer EE. Factors in the production and growth of tumor metastases. J Med Res 1913;28:309–32, 301.
3. Chiarella P, Bruzzo J, Meiss RP, et al. Concomitant tumor resistance. Cancer Lett 2012;324:133–41.
4. Benzekry S, Lamont C, Barbolosi D, et al. Mathematical modeling of tumor-tumor distant interactions supports a systemic control of tumor growth. Cancer Res 2017;77:5183–93.
5. Wang ZY, Mei J, Gao YS, et al. Primary tumorectomy promotes angiogenesis and pulmonary metastasis in osteosarcoma-bearing nude mice. Acta Cir Bras 2013; 28:190–4.
6. Kaya M, Wada T, Nagoya S, et al. Prevention of postoperative progression of pulmonary metastases in osteosarcoma by antiangiogenic therapy using endostatin. J Orthopaedic Sci 2007;12:562–7.
7. Ikeda M, Furukawa H, Imamura H, et al. Surgery for gastric cancer increases plasma levels of vascular endothelial growth factor and von Willebrand factor. Gastric Cancer 2002;5:137–41.
8. Belizon A, Balik E, Feingold DL, et al. Major abdominal surgery increases plasma levels of vascular endothelial growth factor: open more so than minimally invasive methods. Ann Surg 2006;244:792–8.

9. Lacy AM, García-Valdecasas JC, Delgado S, et al. Laparoscopy-assisted colectomy versus open colectomy for treatment of non-metastatic colon cancer: a randomised trial. Lancet 2002;359:2224–9.

10. Da Costa ML, Redmond P, Bouchier-Hayes DJ. The effect of laparotomy and laparoscopy on the establishment of spontaneous tumor metastases. Surgery 1998; 124:516–25.

11. Dubowitz JA, Sloan EK, Riedel BJ. Implicating anaesthesia and the perioperative period in cancer recurrence and metastasis. Clin Exp Metastasis 2018;35: 347–58.

12. Wigmore TJ, Mohammed K, Jhanji S. Long-term survival for patients undergoing volatile versus IV anesthesia for cancer surgery: a retrospective analysis. Anesthesiology 2016;124:69–79.

13. Schlagenhauff B, Ellwanger U, Breuninger H, et al. Prognostic impact of the type of anaesthesia used during the excision of primary cutaneous melanoma. Melanoma Res 2000;10:165–9.

14. Exadaktylos AK, Buggy DJ, Moriarty DC, et al. Can anesthetic technique for primary breast cancer surgery affect recurrence or metastasis? Anesthesiology 2006;105:660–4.

15. Hiller JG, Hacking MB, Link EK, et al. Perioperative epidural analgesia reduces cancer recurrence after gastro-oesophageal surgery. Acta Anaesthesiol Scand 2014;58:281–90.

16. Ciepluch BJ, Wilson-Robles HM, Pashmakova MB, et al. Long-term postoperative effects of administration of allogeneic blood products in 104 dogs with hemangiosarcoma. Vet Surg 2018;47:1039–45.

17. Miyata T, Kodama T, Honma R, et al. Influence of general anesthesia with isoflurane following propofol-induction on natural killer cell cytotoxic activities of peripheral blood lymphocytes in dogs. J Vet Med Sci 2013;75:917–21.

18. Aich A, Gupta P, Gupta K. Could perioperative opioid use increase the risk of cancer progression and metastases? Int Anesthesiol Clin 2016;54:e1–16.

19. Yang W, Cai J, Zabkiewicz C, et al. The effects of anesthetics on recurrence and metastasis of cancer, and clinical implications. World J Oncol 2017;8:63–70.

20. Mathew B, Lennon FE, Siegler J, et al. Novel role of the mu opioid receptor in lung cancer progression: a laboratory study. Anesth Analg 2011;112:558–67.

21. Farooqui M, Li Y, Rogers T, et al. COX-2 inhibitor celecoxib prevents chronic morphine-induced promotion of angiogenesis, tumour growth, metastasis and mortality, without compromising analgesia. Br J Cancer 2007;97:1523–31.

22. Vallejo R, de Leon-Casasola O, Benyamin R. Opioid therapy and immunosuppression: a review. Am J Ther 2004;11:354–65.

23. Shao YJ, Liu WS, Guan BQ, et al. Contribution of opiate analgesics to the development of infections in advanced cancer patients. Clin J Pain 2017;33:295–9.

24. Fecho K, Maslonek KA, Dykstra LA, et al. Evidence for sympathetic and adrenal involvement in the immunomodulatory effects of acute morphine treatment in rats. J Pharmacol Exp Ther 1996;277:633–45.

25. Saurer TB, Carrigan KA, Ijames SG, et al. Suppression of natural killer cell activity by morphine is mediated by the nucleus accumbens shell. J Neuroimmunol 2006; 173:3–11.

26. Saurer TB, Ijames SG, Lysle DT. Neuropeptide Y Y1 receptors mediate morphine-induced reductions of natural killer cell activity. J Neuroimmunol 2006;177:18–26.

27. Boland JW, Pockley AG. Influence of opioids on immune function in patients with cancer pain: from bench to bedside. Br J Pharmacol 2018;175:2726–36.

28. Kraus J. Regulation of mu-opioid receptors by cytokines. Front Biosci (Schol Ed) 2009;1:164–70.
29. Kraus J, Borner C, Giannini E, et al. The role of nuclear factor kappaB in tumor necrosis factor-regulated transcription of the human mu-opioid receptor gene. Mol Pharmacol 2003;64:876–84.
30. Lee BM, Singh Ghotra V, Karam JA, et al. Regional anesthesia/analgesia and the risk of cancer recurrence and mortality after prostatectomy: a meta-analysis. Pain Manag 2015;5:387–95.
31. Singleton PA, Moss J. Effect of perioperative opioids on cancer recurrence: a hypothesis. Future Oncol 2010;6:1237–42.
32. Gupta K, Kshirsagar S, Chang L, et al. Morphine stimulates angiogenesis by activating proangiogenic and survival-promoting signaling and promotes breast tumor growth. Cancer Res 2002;62:4491–8.
33. Bortsov AV, Millikan RC, Belfer I, et al. mu-Opioid receptor gene A118G polymorphism predicts survival in patients with breast cancer. Anesthesiology 2012;116: 896–902.
34. Machado MC, da Costa-Neto JM, Portela RD, et al. The effect of naltrexone as a carboplating chemotherapy-assocaited drug on the immune response, quality of life and survival of dogs with mammary carcinoma. PLoS One 2018;13(10): e0204830.
35. Plein LM, Rittner HL. Opioids and the immune system - friend or foe. Br J Pharmacol 2018;175:2717–25.
36. Tedore T. Regional anaesthesia and analgesia: relationship to cancer recurrence and survival. Br J Anaesth 2015;115(Suppl 2):ii34–45.
37. Franchi S, Panerai AE, Sacerdote P. Buprenorphine ameliorates the effect of surgery on hypothalamus-pituitary-adrenal axis, natural killer cell activity and metastatic colonization in rats in comparison with morphine or fentanyl treatment. Brain Behav Immun 2007;21:767–74.
38. Sacerdote P, Manfredi B, Mantegazza P, et al. Antinociceptive and immunosuppressive effects of opiate drugs: a structure-related activity study. Br J Pharmacol 1997;121:834–40.
39. Doornebal CW, Vrijland K, Hau CS, et al. Morphine does not facilitate breast cancer progression in two preclinical mouse models for human invasive lobular and HER2(+) breast cancer. Pain 2015;156:1424–32.
40. Juneja R. Opioids and cancer recurrence. Curr Opin Support Palliat Care 2014;8: 91–101.
41. KuKanich B, Lascelles BD, Papich MG. Pharmacokinetics of morphine and plasma concentrations of morphine-6-glucuronide following morphine administration to dogs. J Vet Pharmacol Ther 2005;28:371–6.
42. King C, Finley B, Franklin R. The glucuronidation of morphine by dog liver microsomes: identification of morphine-6-O-glucuronide. Drug Metab Dispos 2000;28: 661–3.

Antiinflammatory Drugs

Beatriz Monteiro, DVM, Paulo V. Steagall, MV, MS, PhD*

KEYWORDS

- Analgesia • Dipyrone • Grapiprant • Acetaminophen • Paracetamol • Metamizole
- Nonsteroidal antiinflammatory drugs • Pain

KEY POINTS

- NSAIDs are excellent analgesics that should always be considered for perioperative pain management including pharmacologic and non-pharmacologic therapies, unless otherwise contraindicated. The risk of NSAIDs-induced adverse-effects is minimized by performing a judicious selection of patients, continuous monitoring and careful drug administration.
- Grapiprant is an anti-inflammatory used for the management of canine osteoarthritis. Concurrent administration with other NSAID or corticosteroids should be avoided.
- Paracetamol is contraindicated in cats. In dogs, its use remains mostly anecdotal as few studies have been performed.
- Metamizole is considered an atypical NSAID that seems to be effective in dogs undergoing surgery. Its efficacy in cats remains unknown.
- Corticosteroids have potent anti-inflammatory and immunosuppressive properties but are not considered analgesic drugs.

INTRODUCTION

This article highlights the role of drugs with antiinflammatory effects in the treatment of acute pain and as alternatives to opioids in small animal anesthesia. These drugs act on different pathways of the arachidonic acid cascade (**Fig. 1**). Depending on the type, level, and source of pain, they can be used as a sole agent or in combination with other pharmacologic and nonpharmacologic therapies. There is a strong body of evidence for nonsteroidal antiinflammatory drug (NSAID) use regarding analgesic efficacy and safety profile and this information is presented here, with emphasis on their potential adverse effects. It is beyond the scope of this article to provide an extensive literature review on NSAIDs.

There has been an emerging interest in using metamizole (dipyrone) in dogs and cats, and acetaminophen (paracetamol) in dogs only, as part of a multimodal

Disclosures: None.
Department of Clinical Sciences, Faculty of Veterinary Medicine, Université de Montréal, 3200 rue Sicotte, Saint Hyacinthe, Quebec J2S 2M2, Canada
* Corresponding author.
E-mail address: paulo.steagall@umontreal.ca

Vet Clin Small Anim 49 (2019) 993–1011
https://doi.org/10.1016/j.cvsm.2019.07.009
0195-5616/19/© 2019 Elsevier Inc. All rights reserved.

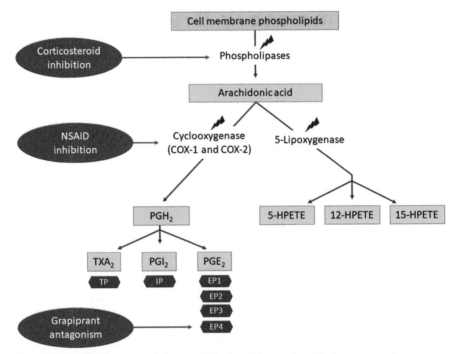

Fig. 1. A simplified version of the arachidonic acid cascade with focus on cyclooxygenase (COX)-dependent prostaglandin production. Corticosteroids act by inhibiting the action of phospholipase enzymes early in the cascade. Nonsteroidal antiinflammatory drugs (NSAIDs) act by inhibiting COX-1 and COX-2 enzymes with consequent inhibition of prostaglandin biosynthesis. Grapiprant is an antagonist of the prostaglandin E2 receptor 4 (EP4). EP1 to EP4, prostaglandin E2 receptors; HPETE, hydroperoxyeicosatetraenate; IP, prostacyclin receptor; PGE_2, prostaglandin E2; PGH_2, prostaglandin H2; PGI_2, prostacyclin; TP, thromboxane receptor; TXA_2, thromboxane.

analgesia regimen, and often in combination with NSAIDs or other nonopioid analgesics for treatment of acute pain. The evidence and recommendations for clinical use for these two drugs are presented in this article.

The misconception on the use of corticosteroids in pain management is a critical issue. Despite their robust antiinflammatory effects, these drugs are not considered conventional analgesics. Their controversies and adverse effects are discussed in the context of acute pain management. In addition, the article presents a summary of evidence for grapiprant, an antagonist of EP4 prostaglandin receptors (see **Fig. 1**) that is approved for the treatment of canine osteoarthritis in several countries but could have a potential role in acute pain management.

NONSTEROIDAL ANTIINFLAMMATORY DRUGS
Mechanism of Action

NSAIDs inhibit expression of cyclooxygenase (COX) enzymes on cell membranes.[1] These enzymes are essential in the biosynthesis of several prostaglandins from the arachidonic acid (see **Fig. 1**). There are at least 2 COX isoforms (COX-1 and COX-2). By inhibiting specific COX enzymes, NSAIDs inhibit the biosynthesis of prostaglandins responsible for different biological and homeostasis functions.

COX-1 is constitutively expressed in many cells. Via prostaglandin biosynthesis, COX-1 is involved with the maintenance of physiologic functions such as vascular homeostasis via thromboxane and prostacyclin production, gastroprotection via secretion of gastric mucous and production of bicarbonate, and renal perfusion (especially under hypotensive conditions).

The COX-2 isoform is primarily released after tissue injury. Via prostaglandin biosynthesis, it is responsible for the production of inflammatory mediators such as endotoxins, cytokines, and growth factors.[2] These mediators participate in the inflammatory response to tissue injury characterized by the cardinal signs of inflammation (pain, heat, redness, swelling, and loss of function). Pain results from the sensitization of peripheral nociceptors by these mediators (ie, transduction) and consequent transmission of the nociceptive input to the spinal cord. The constant and amplified nociceptive input from the periphery to the spinal cord can further result in central sensitization.[3] COX-2 can also play a constitutive role in neural, reproductive, and renal tissues and in ulcer repair.

NSAIDs inhibit the activity of COX enzymes, impairing normal homeostasis at some level, and resulting in the development of adverse effects. The risk of NSAID-induced adverse effects exists even when using preferential or selective COX-2 inhibitors (**Box 1**).

Facts

NSAIDs are metabolized primarily by the liver via glucuronidation in most species. Cats have deficient hepatic glucuronidation and are potentially more susceptible to NSAID-induced adverse effects. However, there are studies supporting the long-term administration of NSAIDs in cats.[4,5]

In the perioperative setting, NSAIDs are safely administered to dogs and cats for the control of inflammation and postoperative pain when contraindications are respected. In cats, these drugs are often administered for several days after surgery, something that would be considered off-label in many countries.[6-9] In addition, the metabolism of some NSAIDs, such as meloxicam, involves oxidative pathways in this species and do not rely on glucuronidation.[10]

NSAIDs are excreted predominantly via the biliary route (fecal) and urine. They accumulate in inflammatory exudates and for this reason intervals of administration are normally every 24 hours despite their short half-lives. The efficacy produced by different NSAIDs is equivalent independently of COX selectivity; however, the safety profile might change according to the drug, doses, intervals and routes of administration,

---

Box 1
The safety of nonsteroidal antiinflammatory drugs is not a simple matter of cyclooxygenase selectivity

It is misleading to consider that the type of COX inhibition (ie, COX-2 selectivity and/or COX-1 sparing) is the only factor regulating NSAID safety. Both COX-1 and COX-2 have physiologic functions that are impaired during NSAID therapy. Any NSAID has the potential to cause adverse effects and contraindications must be respected before drug administration. However, preferential and selective COX-2 inhibitors have a superior safety profile compared with nonselective COX inhibitors.

Data from Luna SPL, Basílio AC, Steagall PVM, et al. Evaluation of adverse effects of long-term oral administration of carprofen, etodolac, flunixin meglumine, ketoprofen, and meloxicam in dogs. *Am J Vet Res.* 2007;68(3):258-264. https://doi.org/10.2460/ajvr.68.3.258.

and species. **Table 1** describes indications and recommendations for dosing and administration of contemporary NSAIDs in Canada and in the United States.

Timing of Administration

The timing of NSAID administration in the perioperative period is a subject of controversy. It is generally accepted that preventive analgesia provides optimal treatment of pain (**Box 2**).[11]

It is arguable that preemptive administration of analgesics (ie, before tissue injury) may maximize the benefits of NSAIDs.[7] For example, the administration of an NSAID after anesthetic induction allows time for the drug to take effect (ie, onset of action) during surgery. In this case, patients may benefit from the antiinflammatory, analgesic, and antipyretic effects of NSAIDs as soon as they are extubated, perhaps helping with a comfortable recovery, in addition to decreasing peripheral nociceptive input to the spinal cord. Studies have shown that healthy dogs can tolerate preemptive administration of NSAIDs, especially if fluid therapy is administered and blood pressure is monitored and maintained within accepted physiologic values.[12–16] The administration of carprofen,[12] meloxicam,[14] or tepoxalin[16] during hypotensive states did not result in clinically important renal adverse effects in healthy anesthetized dogs. However, if there is a concern about the safety of preemptive administration of NSAIDs considering the risk of intraoperative bleeding, hypotension, hypovolemia, and renal hypoperfusion, these drugs should be administered toward the end of the surgical procedure, or at extubation. The risks and benefits of timing of NSAID administration should be evaluated on a case-by-case basis using clinical judgment.

Route of Administration

Most NSAIDs have good palatability and bioavailability after oral administration. Therefore, they are commonly injected parenterally in the perioperative period followed by oral administration in the postoperative period (ie, hospital or home environment), which facilitates treatment compliance. Injectable formulations are commonly given via subcutaneous or intravenous (IV) routes of administration depending on label recommendations (see **Table 1**; **Table 2**). In normothermic patients, peak plasma concentrations of carprofen were higher after oral compared with subcutaneous administration; however, total drug exposure and overall effects were bioequivalent.[17] To the authors' knowledge, similar studies have not been performed in patients with hypothermia with significant peripheral vasoconstriction in which drug absorption/effect could be compromised. Some investigators have speculated that these drugs should then be administered intravenously and slowly in cases of postoperative hypothermia. This method would avoid the aforementioned potential pharmacokinetic-pharmacodynamic issues related to body temperature.

Adverse Effects

Potential adverse effects are based on the rationale of prostaglandin inhibition and include gastrointestinal irritation, protein-losing enteropathy, renal damage, and prolonged bleeding time by prevention of platelet aggregation (**Box 3**).

NSAIDs may produce gastrointestinal changes, including anorexia, diarrhea, and vomiting (**Fig. 2**).[23] The potential for NSAID-induced adverse effects should be clearly communicated to owners; treatment should be immediately stopped if patients become anorexic. NSAID therapy is the most common predisposing factor for gastrointestinal ulceration because of inadvertent administration of human-approved NSAID formulations to companion animals.[24] Ulceration and perforation are usually associated with inappropriate administration, including the concomitant use of a second

Table 1
Label indications and recommendations for commonly used nonsteroidal antiinflammatory drugs in Canada and United States for canine acute pain management

NSAID	Country	Formulation	Recommendation for Dosage and Administration	Indications
Carprofen	Canada	Injectable solution	• 4.4 mg/kg SC every 24 h • Administer approximately 2 h before surgery and once daily thereafter, as needed, for a maximum of 3 consecutive days postoperatively	For the control of postoperative pain associated with soft tissue and orthopedic surgeries in dogs
		Chewable tablets	• 4.4 mg/kg PO every 24 h • May be fed by hand or placed on food	For the relief of pain and inflammation in dogs. Shown to be clinically effective for the control of postoperative pain following orthopedic and soft tissue surgery, in dogs
	United States	Injectable solution	• 4.4 mg/kg SC every 24 h or 2.2 mg/kg SC every 12 h • Administer approximately 2 h before the procedure	For the control of postoperative pain associated with soft tissue and orthopedic surgeries in dogs
		Caplets/chewable tablets	• 4.4 mg/kg PO every 24 h or 2.2 mg/kg PO every 12 h • Administer approximately 2 h before the procedure • May be fed by hand or placed on food	For the control of postoperative pain associated with soft tissue and orthopedic surgeries in dogs
Deracoxib	Canada	Tablets	• Orthopedic surgery: 3–4 mg/kg PO every 24 h as required, for a maximum of 7 d • Dental surgery: 1–2 mg/kg PO every 24 h for a maximum of 3 d • Postprandial administration is preferred	For the relief of pain and inflammation associated with orthopedic surgery; for the relief of postoperative pain and inflammation associated with dental surgery
	United States	Chewable tablets	• Orthopedic surgery: 3–4 mg/kg PO every 24 h, as needed, for a maximum of 7 d • Dental surgery: 1–2 mg/kg PO every 24 h for a maximum of 3 d • The first dose should be given approximately 1 h before dental surgery • Postprandial administration is preferred	For the control of pain and inflammation associated with orthopedic surgery and dental surgery in dogs

(continued on next page)

Table 1
(continued)

NSAID	Country	Formulation	Recommendation for Dosage and Administration	Indications
Firocoxib	United States	Chewable tablets	• 5 mg/kg PO every 24 h as needed for a maximum of 3 d • Administer approximately 2 hours before surgery with or without food • Use the lowest effective dose for the shortest duration consistent with individual response	For the control of postoperative pain and inflammation associated with soft tissue and orthopedic surgery in dogs
Meloxicam	Canada	Oral suspension	• 0.2 mg/kg PO once, followed by 0.1 mg/kg PO every 24 h • Should be administered mixed with food	For the alleviation of inflammation and pain in acute musculoskeletal disorders
		Injectable solution	• 0.2 mg/kg IV or SC once before surgery	For the alleviation of inflammation and pain in acute musculoskeletal disorders and for the control of perioperative pain following orthopedic and soft tissue surgery
		Chewable tablets	• 0.2 mg/kg PO once, followed by 0.1 mg/kg every 24 h	For the alleviation of inflammation and pain in acute musculoskeletal disorders
Robenacoxib	Canada	Injectable	• Orthopedic and soft tissue surgery: 2 mg/kg SC once • Administer approximately 30 min before the start of surgery, around the time of induction of general anesthesia • As an adjuvant in soft tissue surgery: 2 mg/kg SC every 24 h for a maximum of 3 d • Administer approximately 30–45 min before the start of surgery as the preanesthetic agents are given • After surgery treatment may be given via injection or interchanged with the oral tablet • If subsequent doses are given by subcutaneous injection, different sites for each injection should be used	For the control of pain and inflammation associated with orthopedic or soft tissue surgery; as an adjunctive medication in the control of postoperative pain and inflammation associated with soft tissue surgery

	Tablets	• 2 mg/kg PO every 24 h for a maximum of 3 d • The first dose should be administered approximately 30–45 min (without food) before the start of surgery, at the same time as the preanesthetic agents • After surgery, treatment may be continued with tablets or injection • If subsequent doses are given by subcutaneous injection, different sites for each injection should be used	As an adjunctive medication in the control of postoperative pain and inflammation associated with soft tissue surgery in dogs ≥2.5 kg and ≥4 mo of age
United States	Injectable solution	• 2 mg/kg SC every 24 h for a maximum of 3 d • The first dose should be administered approximately 45 min before surgery, at the same time as the preanesthetic agents • Subsequent doses can be given via subcutaneous injection, or interchanged with the oral tablets	For the control of postoperative pain and inflammation associated with soft tissue surgery in dogs ≥4 mo of age
	Tablets	• 2 mg/kg PO every 24 h for a maximum of 3 d • Administer the first dose approximately 45 min before surgery, at the same time as preanesthetic agents • Subsequent doses can be given via oral tablet or interchanged with SC injection	For the control of postoperative pain and inflammation associated with soft tissue surgery in dogs ≥2.5 kg and ≥4 mo of age

Label information was collected from the manufacturer's Web site. Minor editions were performed for the purpose of this article. This table is meant to serve as a guide for general use. Veterinarians are invited to contact the NSAID manufacturers for detailed and updated information on label indications, dosage, and administration.

Abbreviations: IV, intravenous; PO, orally; SC, subcutaneous.

Box 2
Preventive and preemptive analgesia, and the administration of nonsteroidal antiinflammatory drugs

- Preventive analgesia includes the administration of perioperative analgesic techniques (ie, multimodal analgesia) leading to reduced postoperative pain scores and analgesic requirements.

- Preemptive analgesia (ie, administration of analgesics before tissue injury) is a technique of preventive analgesia. However, this terminology has been used less frequently in the recent literature because its benefits compared with postoperative administration of analgesics have not always been shown in human studies.

- The amount of intraoperative tissue damage and/or the presence of preoperative pain can influence the severity and duration of postoperative pain. NSAIDs play a major role in preventive analgesia in companion animals. They should preferably be administered in combination with local anesthetic techniques and other nonopioid analgesics to minimize postoperative pain as alternatives to opioid analgesia.

NSAID or a corticosteroid, higher than labeled doses, or lack of close patient monitoring.[24–27] For example, the concomitant administration of meloxicam with dexamethasone during 3 days resulted in higher scores of gastrointestinal lesions detected by endoscopy compared with dexamethasone alone.[28]

Adverse effects are also observed more frequently in patients with preexisting conditions (eg, hypovolemia, dehydration) that would normally contraindicate the administration of NSAIDs (**Box 4**).[23] Supportive therapy must be initiated on a case-by-case basis, including fluid therapy and administration of gastroprotectants.

The NSAID-associated renal adverse effects are generally difficult to assess in the clinical setting unless changes are severe and renal disease is significant. Monitoring creatinine and blood urea nitrogen (BUN) is not a sensitive means of assessing early kidney disease. NSAID-induced renal adverse effects have not been reported in the canine and feline literature except when these drugs were combined with nephrotoxic agents. As previously mentioned, clinically detectable adverse effects in healthy dogs being administered NSAIDs and submitted to general anesthesia and hypotension were not observed in previous studies.[12,14,16] It should be noted that the renal effects of NSAIDs in dogs and cats with comorbidities and hypotension during general anesthesia remain unknown. Therefore, patients should be appropriately screened for NSAID administration. For example, increases in creatinine level in a young and healthy patient may simply indicate dehydration caused by transport and long-term fasting. Withholding an NSAID in this case without any other clear evidence of contra-indication could lead to pain and suffering in the postoperative period. Fluid therapy should be administered and the concentrations of BUN and creatinine, and BUN/creatinine ratio, should be reevaluated for a final decision on NSAID administration.

Specific Information on the Administration of Nonsteroidal Antiinflammatory Drugs in Cats

- The efficacy and safety of meloxicam and robenacoxib for the treatment of feline acute pain has been shown in different studies using different doses, routes, and intervals of administration.[4,30]

- Meloxicam was administered for up to 7 days in healthy cats with experimentally induced reduced renal mass without changes in glomerular filtration rate, creatinine levels, or urine protein/creatinine ratio.[31]

Table 2
Label indications for commonly used nonsteroidal antiinflammatory drugs in Canada and United States for feline acute pain management

NSAID	Country	Formulation	Recommendation for Dosage and Administration	Indications
Meloxicam	Canada	Injectable solution	• 0.2 mg/kg SC once before surgery • Give the lowest effective dose • The use of parenteral fluids during surgery should be considered to reduce the risk of renal toxicity when using NSAIDs perioperatively	For the control of perioperative pain following orthopedic and soft tissue surgery
		Oral suspension	• After initial treatment with injectable meloxicam, continue treatment 24 h later with 0.05 mg/kg PO (oral suspension) every 24 h for up to 2 d	For the alleviation of inflammation and pain following surgery such as onychectomy, ovariohysterectomy, or castration, or associated with acute, mild to moderate musculoskeletal disorders in cats
	United States	Injectable solution	• 0.3 mg/kg SC once • Use of additional meloxicam or other NSAIDs is contraindicated	For the control of postoperative pain and inflammation associated with orthopedic surgery, ovariohysterectomy and castration when administered before surgery
Robenacoxib	Canada	Injectable	• 2 mg/kg SC every 24 h for a maximum of 3 d • Administer approximately 30 min before the start of surgery, around the time the preanesthetic agents are given • After surgery, treatment may be continued using injectable or oral formulations • If subsequent doses are given by subcutaneous injection, different sites for each injection should be used	As an adjunctive medication in the control of postoperative pain and inflammation associated with onychectomy, ovariohysterectomy, and castration in cats

(continued on next page)

Table 2
(continued)

NSAID	Country	Formulation	Recommendation for Dosage and Administration	Indications
		Tablets	• Cat bites and scratches and musculoskeletal injuries: 1–2.4 mg/kg PO every 24 h for a maximum of 6 d • Postoperative pain: 1–2.4 mg/kg PO every 24 h for a maximum of 3 d • The first dose should be administered approximately 30 min (without food) before the start of the surgery, around the time of induction of general anesthesia • After surgery, treatment may be continued with tablets or injection at the respective label recommended dose • If subsequent doses are given by subcutaneous injection, different sites for each injection should be used	For the relief of acute pain and inflammation associated with cat bites and scratches with and without abscesses and musculoskeletal injuries such as sprains and strains; as an adjunctive medication, in the control of postoperative pain and inflammation associated with onychectomy, ovariohysterectomy, and castration
	United States	Injectable solution	• 2 mg/kg SC every 24 h for a maximum of 3 d • Use the lowest effective dose for the shortest duration consistent with individual response	For the control of postoperative pain and inflammation associated with orthopedic surgery, ovariohysterectomy, and castration in cats ≥4 mo of age

Label information was collected from the manufacturer's Web site. Minor editions were performed for the purpose of this article. This table is meant to serve as a guide for general use. Veterinarians are invited to contact the manufacturers of NSAIDs for detailed and updated information on label indications, dosage, and administration.

Abbreviations: PO, by mouth; SC, subcutaneous.

> **Box 3**
> **Do nonsteroidal antiinflammatory drugs and acetylsalicylic acid make dogs and cats bleed intraoperatively?**
>
> - The activation of COX-1 leads to the production of thromboxane A2 and consequent platelet aggregation and vasoconstriction, whereas the activation of COX-2 leads to the production of prostacyclin and consequent anticoagulation effects and vasodilation.
> - The balance between the activity of both COX enzymes promotes hemostasis (ie, avoids thrombosis and uncontrolled bleeding). This balance could be disrupted after the administration of NSAIDs or acetylsalicylic acid.
> - Acetylsalicylic acid binds irreversibly to the COX complex and may impair platelet aggregation for the duration of the platelet lifespan. NSAIDs could potentially impair platelet aggregation during drug administration. However, these effects are reversible once therapy is stopped.
> - Studies performed on dogs undergoing surgery and being administered ketoprofen[19] or meloxicam[20] preemptively found decreases in platelet aggregation[19] and small increases in activated partial thromboplastin time[20] after surgery. Nevertheless, buccal mucosal bleeding time remained unchanged in both studies and, despite observed changes, values were usually within normal limits.
> - Studies performed to evaluate the hemostatic effects of different NSAIDs generally showed minimal changes in the coagulation profile. The clinical significance of these findings are likely irrelevant in healthy dogs.[18,21,22]
> - NSAIDs are contraindicated in patients with anemia and coagulopathies.
>
> *Data from* Refs.[18–22]

- Different clinical trials have shown that meloxicam, tolfenamic acid, ketoprofen, and robenacoxib are mostly similar in terms of analgesic efficacy in postoperative pain (ie, orthopedic and soft tissue surgery) or acute pain disorders (ie, acute musculoskeletal muscle disorders).[6,9,32–34] Palatability is superior with meloxicam and robenacoxib compared with ketoprofen or tolfenamic acid, which is important in cats, especially for the treatment of persistent postsurgical pain.[6,32,33]

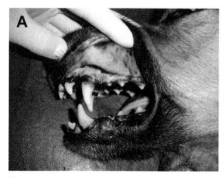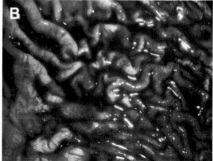

Fig. 2. Inappropriate NSAID administration can result in severe gastrointestinal adverse effects. This dog was continually administered a NSAID in the presence of anorexia, vomiting and diarrhead, and died shortly after presentation. (*A*) Necropsy findings revealed markedly pale and icteric mucous membranes with signs of hepatic insufficiency and (*B*) severe gastrointestinal hemorrhage.

Box 4
Relative contraindications for nonsteroidal antiinflammatory drug administration

- History of gastrointestinal disease
- NSAID intolerance[a]
- Uncontrolled renal or hepatic disease
- Anemia
- Coagulopathy
- Hypovolemia or dehydration
- Hypotension
- Concurrent corticosteroid administration
- Close temporal administration of other NSAIDs[b]

[a] Intolerance to one NSAID does not necessarily preclude the animal from treatment with a different NSAID after a washout period.
[b] The ideal washout period between 2 different NSAIDs is unknown for both dogs and cats. Clinical experience shows that 3 to 5 days is acceptable in patients without clinical signs.[23,29] Other analgesics should be administered for pain management during the washout period.
Data from Monteiro-Steagall BP, Steagall PVM, Lascelles BDX. Systematic Review of Nonsteroidal Anti-Inflammatory Drug-Induced Adverse Effects in Dogs. J Vet Intern Med. 2013;27(5):1011-1019. https://doi.org/10.1111/jvim.12127; and Lascelles BDX, McFarland JM, Swann H. Guidelines for safe and effective use of NSAIDs in dogs. Vet Ther. 2005;6(3):237-251.

- Readers should be aware of several study limitations within these clinical trials and interpret the results with caution. The specific end points in some of these studies have never been validated, and veterinarians and owners are not always adequately trained in assessing acute pain in feline patients. For example, it is surprising that none of the cats required rescue analgesia postoperatively in some of these studies.[8] The lack of pain recognition in studies with cats has previously been criticized in the literature.[35]
- Robenacoxib should be preferentially administered by IV or subcutaneous injection in the perioperative period. If administered orally, the feeding schedule can influence bioavailability and maximum plasma concentrations; thus, the drug should be administered orally after food withholding or with a small amount of food.[36]
- Meloxicam and robenacoxib have undergone several investigations for the treatment of long-term pain in both the research and clinical settings, and were shown to be safe and palatable for long-term administration, including in cats with osteoarthritis and stable chronic kidney disease.[4,5,37–39] The effects of NSAIDs in cats with chronic kidney disease undergoing anesthesia for surgery with concomitant hypotension, hypovolemia, etc., remain unknown. Thus, the perioperative administration of NSAIDs to cats with stable chronic kidney disease should be judicious. The concept of minimal effective dosage should always be applied when dosing NSAIDs and, ideally, cats should be drinking and eating normally in the postoperative period before drug administration. A review on the use of NSAIDs in cats with concomitant chronic pain and chronic kidney disease is available elsewhere.[40]

GRAPIPRANT
Mechanism of Action

Arachidonic acid is converted by COX enzymes into prostanoids, including prostaglandin E2. Prostaglandin E2 activates specific receptors, including the EP4.[41] EP4 is one of the receptors involved in the prostaglandin E2–induced inflammation and sensitization of sensory neurons. Piprants are EP4 prostaglandin receptor antagonists (**Fig. 1**). Therefore, piprants produce analgesic and antiinflammatory effects by selectively inhibiting a single prostanoid receptor without inhibiting other homeostatic functions by prostaglandins.[41]

Grapiprant is a piprant that selectively blocks the EP4 receptor; it is licensed (2 mg/kg orally every 24 hours) in various countries for management of pain and inflammation associated with canine osteoarthritis. The drug has shown a good safety profile in dogs and cats.[42–44]

It may be common for dogs that are being treated with grapiprant for osteoarthritis to have to undergo painful surgical procedures. Concomitant use of grapiprant and NSAIDs or corticosteroids has not been studied and the combinations should be avoided. Veterinarians should probably continue the administration of grapiprant for postoperative pain, bearing in mind that the administration would be off label because studies using grapiprant for the control of postoperative pain have not been published at the time of writing. Potential adverse effects may occur after the administration of grapiprant.

Scientific Evidence

- In a safety and toxicology study involving research beagles, vomiting and soft stools were more commonly observed in dogs receiving grapiprant via oral gavage (50 mg/kg every 24 hours for 9 months) compared with placebo.[43] No drug-related effects on liver enzyme levels, BUN levels, creatinine values, or platelet function were detected. Note that this was a 25-fold increase in labeled doses for oral administration.
- In a prospective, randomized, masked, placebo-controlled, multicenter clinical trial including 285 dogs, treatment with grapiprant (2 mg/kg orally every 24 h) for 28 days improved pain scores based on the Canine Brief Pain Inventory when compared with placebo. Treatment was generally well tolerated but the frequency of adverse effects was higher in treated versus placebo-treated dogs.[42] Most common adverse effects included vomiting, diarrhea or soft stools, and anorexia or decreased appetite. These effects were generally mild and resolved without treatment.[42]
- The safety profile of grapiprant was investigated in research cats. No clinically significant adverse effects were detected on body weight, food consumption, clinicopathologic values, or necropsy findings.[44] Grapiprant is not labeled for use in cats and its efficacy remains to be investigated.

ACETAMINOPHEN (PARACETAMOL)
Mechanism of Action

Acetaminophen produces analgesic and antipyretic effects but has weak antiinflammatory activity. It inhibits prostaglandin E2 synthesis in the central nervous system. The presence of COX-3, a subform of COX-1, has been found in the canine and human cerebral cortex.[45] It has been suggested that acetaminophen and metamizole, and potentially some NSAIDs, selectively inhibit COX-3 expression and consequent prostaglandin E2 synthesis, implicating a central mechanism of these drugs as opposed to the primarily peripheral action of most NSAIDs.[45,46]

Clinical Use

Acetaminophen is contraindicated in cats. In dogs, it has been used for the management of acute pain of traumatic origin and after surgery in the United Kingdom but also for the treatment of chronic pain as part of a multimodal approach. Anecdotally, it has also been used for its analgesic properties during the washout period when switching between different NSAIDs. However, there is a lack of scientific evidence for the administration of acetaminophen in dogs. Based on the data available so far and lack of antinociceptive and analgesic effects, there is no evidence to support its use in dogs (discussed later). In humans, the drug is normally administered by the IV or oral routes of administration with good efficacy profile. However, pharmacokinetics and pharmacodynamics are different among species and these data cannot be extrapolated to dogs.

Scientific Evidence

- In a clinical study involving 50 dogs undergoing tibial plateau–leveling osteotomy, the analgesic efficacy of orally administered hydrocodone-acetaminophen (13–18 mg/kg of acetaminophen) was compared with tramadol during the postoperative period. One dose of morphine (0.25–0.5 mg/kg subcutaneously) was also injected shortly after surgery. Regurgitation and drooling were recorded after hydrocodone-acetaminophen. Rescue analgesia was required in 5 out of 19 dogs receiving hydrocodone-acetaminophen and in 7 out of 23 dogs receiving tramadol. The prevalence of treatment failure was considered unacceptable with both treatments.[47] It is not known whether these treatments would provide any analgesic benefit when administered in combination with other analgesics.
- The pharmacokinetics and antinociceptive effects of a combination of orally administered acetaminophen (600 mg; 14.4–23.1 mg/kg) and codeine phosphate (90 mg; 2.1–3.3 mg/kg) were investigated in 6 healthy greyhounds. Antinociception was assessed using an electronic von Frey and no effect of treatment was observed.[48]
- Acetaminophen (10.5 mg/kg mean dose) in combination with codeine (1.43 mg/kg mean dose) is rapidly absorbed and eliminated after oral administration in dogs.[49]
- The pharmacokinetics of acetaminophen were investigated after oral and rectal administration (325 mg; 9.3–13 mg/kg) in healthy and ill hospitalized dogs. Bioavailability was lower after rectal compared with oral administration. For both routes of administration, acetaminophen did not reach or sustain plasma concentrations associated with efficacy in humans.[50] It is unknown whether similar plasma concentrations produce analgesia in dogs.
- Clinical studies using different doses and routes of administration of acetaminophen should be performed in dogs before further indications are recommended.

Safety Profile

Acetaminophen toxicosis can result secondary to hepatotoxicity or methemoglobinemia. In humans, hepatotoxicity is more common, whereas dogs and cats primarily develop methemoglobinemia.[51–54] In dogs, acetaminophen is conjugated with glucuronide and sulfate by transferase enzymes. Cats have deficient glucuronidation and are much more sensite to acetaminophen toxicity. For example, clinical signs of acetaminophen toxicity in dogs generally develop with doses of 150 to 200 mg/kg, whereas, in cats, this can occur with doses of 60 mg/kg. Clinical signs of methemoglobinemia include cyanosis, facial edema, prolapse of conjunctival membranes, brown blood and urine, tachypnea, and dyspnea. Supportive treatment includes fluid therapy, N-acetylcysteine, ascorbic acid, and sodium bicarbonate. For these reasons, acetaminophen is strictly contraindicated in cats.

METAMIZOLE (DIPYRONE)
Mechanism of Action

Metamizole (dipyrone) is considered an atypical NSAID with weak antiinflammatory properties, but potent analgesic effects that are thought to be related mainly via central inhibition of COX-3 enzyme.[45] In humans, it is often used for the management of postoperative pain in cases in which NSAIDs are contraindicated.[55] Opioid and cannabinoid systems are also possible mechanisms related to analgesia.[56]

Clinical Use

Metamizole is not approved for use in companion animals in North America, but it is widely used in South America and some countries in Europe.

Scientific Evidence

- Metamizole was shown to provide adequate postoperative analgesia in dogs undergoing ovariohysterectomy (25–35 mg/kg IV every 8 hours).[57]
- Metamizole alone (25 mg/kg IV administered preoperatively) or in combination with meloxicam reduced the prevalence of rescue analgesia compared with placebo or meloxicam alone in dogs undergoing ovariohysterectomy.[58] Analgesic and antihyperalgesic effects were observed when metamizole and meloxicam were combined.
- The combination of tramadol-metamizole with or without carprofen or meloxicam was well tolerated and clinically effective to treat moderate to severe pain in dogs with cancer.[59]
- In contrast, metamizole (50 mg/kg IV) did not produce antinociception or any anesthetic-sparing effects in dogs undergoing anesthesia with sevoflurane.[60] The investigators questioned the benefits of using metamizole in canine patients.
- The pharmacokinetic profiles of IV and intramuscular (IM) administration of metamizole (25 mg/kg) were comparable; systemic absorption was the least effective after rectal administration in dogs.[61]
- The IV administration of metamizole alone or with meloxicam resulted in decreased platelet aggregation. However, it did not affect thromboelastometry or buccal mucosal bleeding time in healthy conscious dogs.[62]
- The pharmacokinetics of the 2 major metabolites of metamizole (4-methylaminoantipyrine and 4-aminoantipyrine; 25 mg/kg) after IV, IM, and oral administration were studied in cats. Metamizole was converted into its active metabolites similarly to other species.[63] Salivation and vomiting were observed in 4 out of 6 and 2 out of 6 cats after IV and IM administration, respectively.
- The analgesic effects of metamizole in cats remain unknown at the time of writing.

CORTICOSTEROIDS
Mechanism of Action

Glucocorticosteroids are a class of corticosteroids that are largely used for their potent antiinflammatory and immunosuppressive properties in the management of conditions such as hypoadrenocorticism and immune-mediated disorders. These drugs are not considered analgesics and should not be used as alternatives to opioid analgesia. There is little scientific evidence to support their use in the treatment of acute pain based on their efficacy and safety profiles. Their use is severely hampered by the high risk of development of adverse effects. These effects include polyuria and polydipsia, polyphagia, gastrointestinal disorders, iatrogenic hyperadrenocorticism, muscle atrophy, increased risk of infection, and poor wound healing.[64] Glucocorticos-teroids should not be used concomitantly or in close temporal association with NSAIDs because of increased incidence of adverse effects, especially gastrointestinal ulcers.[28] Their high prevalence of adverse effects outweighs their robust antiinflamma-tory effects when used for the treatment of pain.

REFERENCES

1. Flower RJ, Vane JR. Inhibition of prostaglandin synthetase in brain explains the anti-pyretic activity of paracetamol (4-acetamidophenol). Nature 1972;240(5381): 410–1.

2. Kulkarni SK, Jain NK, Singh A. Cyclooxygenase isoenzymes and newer thera-peutic potential for selective COX-2 inhibitors. Methods Find Exp Clin Pharmacol 2000;22(5):291–8.

3. Lees P, Landoni M, Giraudel J, et al. Pharmacodynamics and pharmacokinetics of non steroidal anti-inflammatory drugs in species of veterinary interest.pdf. J Vet Pharmacol Ther 2004;27:479–90.

4. Gunew MN, Menrath VH, Marshall RD. Long-term safety, efficacy and palatability of oral meloxicam at 0.01-0.03 mg/kg for treatment of osteoarthritic pain in cats. J Feline Med Surg 2008;10(3):235–41.

5. King JN, King S, Budsberg SC, et al. Clinical safety of robenacoxib in feline oste-oarthritis: results of a randomized, blinded, placebo-controlled clinical trial. J Feline Med Surg 2016;18(8):632–42.

6. Morton CM, Grant D, Johnston L, et al. Clinical evaluation of meloxicam versus ketoprofen in cats suffering from painful acute locomotor disorders. J Feline Med Surg 2011;13(4):237–43.

7. Ingwersen W, Fox R, Cunningham G, et al. Efficacy and safety of 3 versus 5 days of meloxicam as an analgesic for feline onychectomy and sterilization. Can Vet J 2012;53:257–64.

8. Kamata M, King JN, Seewald W, et al. Comparison of injectable robenacoxib versus meloxicam for peri-operative use in cats: results of a randomised clinical trial. Vet J 2012;193(1):114–8.

9. Speranza C, Schmid V, Giraudel JM, et al. Robenacoxib versus meloxicam for the control of peri-operative pain and inflammation associated with orthopaedic sur-gery in cats: a randomised clinical trial. BMC Vet Res 2015;11(1).

10. Grude P, Guittard J, Garcia C, et al. Excretion mass balance evaluation, metab-olite profile analysis and metabolite identification in plasma and excreta after oral administration of [14C]-meloxicam to the male cat: preliminary study. J Vet Phar-macol Ther 2010;33(4):396–407.

11. Kaye AD, Urman RD, Vadivelu N, et al. Preventive analgesia for postoperative pain control : a broader concept. Local Reg Anesth 2014;7(1):17–22.

12. Boström IM, Nyman GC, Lord PE, et al. Effects of carprofen on renal function and results of serum biochemical and hematologic analyses in anesthetized dogs that had low blood pressure during anesthesia. Am J Vet Res 2002;63(5):712–21.

13. Crandell DE, Mathews KA, Dyson DH. Effect of meloxicam and carprofen on renal function when administered to healthy dogs prior to anesthesia and painful stim-ulation. Am J Vet Res 2004;65(10):1384–90.

14. Boström IM, Nyman G, Hoppe A, et al. Effects of meloxicam on renal function in dogs with hypotension during anaesthesia. Vet Anaesth Analg 2006;33(1):62–9.

15. Frendin JHM, Boström IM, Kampa N, et al. Effects of carprofen on renal function during medetomine-propofol-isoflurane anesthesia in dogs. Am J Vet Res 2006; 67(12):1967–73.

16. Lopes C, Carregaro AB, Freitas GC, et al. Effect of tepoxalin on renal function and hepatic enzymes in dogs exposed to hypotension with isoflurane. Vet Anaesth Analg 2014;41(5):459–67.

17. Clark TP, Chieffo C, Huhn JC, et al. The steady-state pharmacokinetics and bio-equivalence of carprofen administered orally and subcutaneously in dogs. J Vet Pharmacol Ther 2003;26(3):187–92.

18. Luna SPL, Basílio AC, Steagall PVM, et al. Evaluation of adverse effects of long-term oral administration of carprofen, etodolac, flunixin meglumine, ketoprofen, and meloxicam in dogs. Am J Vet Res 2007;68(3):258–64.

19. Lemke KA, Runyon CL, Horney BS. Effects of preoperative administration of ketoprofen on whole blood platelet aggregation, buccal mucosal bleeding time, and hematologic indices in dogs undergoing elective ovariohysterectomy. J Am Vet Med Assoc 2002;220(12):1818–22.

20. Kazakos GM, Papazoglou LG, Rallis T, et al. Effects of meloxicam on the haemostatic profile of dogs undergoing orthopaedic surgery. Vet Rec 2005;157(15): 444–6.

21. Brainard BM, Meredith CP, Callan MB, et al. Changes in platelet function, hemostasis, & PG expression after treatment w/NSAIDs w/various COX selectivities in dogs. Am J Vet Res 2007;68(3):251–7.

22. Blois SL, Allen DG, Wood RD, et al. Effects of aspirin, carprofen, deracoxib, and meloxicam on platelet function and systemic prostaglandin concentrations in healthy dogs. Am J Vet Res 2010;71(3):349–58.

23. Monteiro-Steagall BP, Steagall PVM, Lascelles BDX. Systematic review of nonsteroidal anti-inflammatory drug-induced adverse effects in dogs. J Vet Intern Med 2013;27(5):1011–9.

24. Lascelles BDX, Blikslager AT, Fox SM, et al. Gastrointestinal tract perforation in dogs treated with a selective cyclooxygenase-2 inhibitor: 29 cases (2002-2003). J Am Vet Med Assoc 2005;227(7):1112–7.

25. Jones RD, Baynes RE, Nimitz CT. Nonsteroidal anti-inflammatory drug toxicosis in dogs and cats: 240 cases (1989-1990). J Am Vet Med Assoc 1992;201(3):475–7.

26. Enberg TB, Braun LD, Kuzma AB. Gastrointestinal perforation in five dogs associated with the administration of meloxicam. J Vet Emerg Crit Care 2006;16(1): 34–43.

27. Narita T, Sato R, Motoishi K, et al. The interaction between orally administered non-steroidal anti-inflammatory drugs and prednisolone in healthy dogs. J Vet Med Sci 2007;69(4):353–63.

28. Boston SE, Moens NMM, Kruth SA, et al. Endoscopic evaluation of the gastroduodenal mucosa to determine the safety of short-term concurrent administration of meloxicam and dexamethasone in healthy dogs. Am J Vet Res 2003;64(11): 1369–75.

29. Lascelles BDX, McFarland JM, Swann H. Guidelines for safe and effective use of NSAIDs in dogs. Vet Ther 2005;6(3):237–51.

30. King JN, Hotz R, Reagan EL, et al. Safety of oral robenacoxib in the cat. J Vet Pharmacol Ther 2012;35(3):290–300.

31. Surdyk KK, Brown CA, Brown SA. Evaluation of glomerular filtration rate in cats with reduced renal mass and administered meloxicam and acetylsalicylic acid. Am J Vet Res 2013;74(4):648–51.

32. Benito-de-la-Víbora J, Lascelles BDX, García-Fernández P, et al. Efficacy of tolfenamic acid and meloxicam in the control of postoperative pain following ovariohysterectomy in the cat. Vet Anaesth Analg 2008;35(6):501–10.

33. Murison PJ, Tacke S, Wondratschek C, et al. Postoperative analgesic efficacy of meloxicam compared to tolfenamic acid in cats undergoing orthopaedic surgery. J Small Anim Pract 2010;51(10):526–32.

34. Giraudel JM, Gruet P, Alexander DG, et al. Evaluation of orally administered robenacoxib versus ketoprofen for treatment of acute pain and inflammation associated with musculoskeletal disorders in cats. Am J Vet Res 2010;71(7):710–9.

35. Wareham K, Doit H. Robenacoxib for acute musculoskeletal pain control in cats. Vet Rec 2017;180(15):381–3.

36. King JN, Jung M, Maurer MP, et al. Effects of route of administration and feeding schedule on pharmacokinetics of robenacoxib in cats. Am J Vet Res 2013;74(3): 465–72.

37. Gowan RA, Lingard AE, Johnston L, et al. Retrospective case-control study of the effects of long-term dosing with meloxicam on renal function in aged cats with degenerative joint disease. J Feline Med Surg 2011;13(10):752–61.

38. Gowan RA, Baral RM, Lingard AE, et al. A retrospective analysis of the effects of meloxicam on the longevity of aged cats with and without overt chronic kidney disease. J Feline Med Surg 2012;14(12):876–81.

39. Guillot M, Moreau M, Heit M, et al. Characterization of osteoarthritis in cats and meloxicam efficacy using objective chronic pain evaluation tools. Vet J 2013; 196(3):360–7.

40. Monteiro B, Steagall PVM, Lascelles BDX, et al. Long-term use of non-steroidal anti-inflammatory drugs in cats with chronic kidney disease: from controversy to optimism. J Small Anim Pract 2019;60(8):459–62.

41. Kirkby Shaw K, Rausch-Derra LC, Rhodes L. Grapiprant: an EP4 prostaglandin receptor antagonist and novel therapy for pain and inflammation. Vet Med Sci 2016;2(1):3–9.

42. Rausch-Derra L, Huebner M, Wofford J, et al. A prospective, randomized, masked, placebo-controlled multisite clinical study of Grapiprant, an EP4 prostaglandin receptor antagonist (PRA), in dogs with osteoarthritis. J Vet Intern Med 2016;30(3):756–63.

43. Rausch-Derra LC, Huebner M, Rhodes L. Evaluation of the safety of long-term, daily oral administration of grapiprant, a novel drug for treatment of osteoarthritic pain and inflammation, in healthy dogs. Am J Vet Res 2015;76(10):853–9.

44. Rausch-Derra LC, Rhodes L. Safety and toxicokinetic profiles associated with daily oral administration of grapiprant, a selective antagonist of the prostaglandin E2EP4 receptor, to cats. Am J Vet Res 2016;77(7):688–92.

45. Chandrasekharan NV, Dai H, Roos K, et al. COX-3, a cyclooxygenase-1 variant inhibited by acetaminophen and other analgesic/antipyretic drugs: cloning, structure, and expression. Proc Natl Acad Sci U S A 2002;99(21):13926–31.

46. Botting R, Ayoub SS. COX-3 and the mechanism of action of paracetamol/acetaminophen. Prostaglandins Leukot Essent Fatty Acids 2005;72(2):85–7.

47. Benitez ME, Roush JK, McMurphy R, et al. Clinical efficacy of hydrocodone-acetaminophen and tramadol for control of postoperative pain in dogs following tibial plateau leveling osteotomy. Am J Vet Res 2015;76(9):755–62.

48. KuKanich B. Pharmacokinetics and pharmacodynamics of oral acetaminophen in combination with codeine in healthy Greyhound dogs. J Vet Pharmacol Ther 2016;39(5):514–7.

49. Kukanich B. Pharmacokinetics of acetaminophen, codeine, and the codeine metabolites morphine and codeine-6-glucuronide in healthy Greyhound dogs. J Vet Pharmacol Ther 2009;33(1):15–21.
50. Sikina ER, Bach JF, Lin Z, et al. Bioavailability of suppository acetaminophen in healthy and critically ill dogs. J Vet Pharmacol Ther 2018;41:652–8.
51. MacNaughton S. Acetaminophen toxicosis in a Dalmatian. Can Vet J 2003;44: 142–4.
52. Nielsen L, Shaw M, Morris J. What is your diagnosis? Paracetamol poisoning. J Small Anim Pract 2007;48(2):121–4.
53. McConkey SE, Grant DM, Cribb AE. The role of para-aminophenol in acetaminophen-induced methemoglobinemia in dogs and cats. J Vet Pharmacol Ther 2009;32(6):585–95.
54. Stewart J, Haslam A, Puig J. Pathology in practice. Acetaminophen (paracetamol) toxicosis. J Am Vet Med Assoc 2016;248(9):1009–11.
55. Konijnenbelt-Peters J, van der Heijden C, Ekhart C, et al. Metamizole (Dipyrone) as an alternative agent in postoperative analgesia in patients with contraindications for nonsteroidal anti-inflammatory drugs. Pain Pract 2017;17(3):402–8.
56. Jasiecka A, Maślanka T, Jaroszewski JJ. Pharmacological characteristics of metamizole. Pol J Vet Sci 2014;17(1):207–14.
57. Imagawa VH, Fantoni DT, Tatarunas AC, et al. The use of different doses of metamizol for post-operative analgesia in dogs. Vet Anaesth Analg 2011;38(4): 385–93.
58. Zanuzzo FS, Teixeira-Neto FJ, Teixeira LR, et al. Analgesic and antihyperalgesic effects of dipyrone, meloxicam or a dipyrone-meloxicam combination in bitches undergoing ovariohysterectomy. Vet J 2015;205(1):33–7.
59. Flôr PB, Yazbek KV, Ida KK, et al. Tramadol plus metamizole combined or not with anti-inflammatory drugs is clinically effective for moderate to severe chronic pain treatment in cancer patients. Vet Anaesth Analg 2013;40(3):316–27.
60. Schütter AF, Tünsmeyer J, Kästner SB. Influence of metamizole on 1) minimal alveolar concentration of sevoflurane in dogs and 2) on thermal and mechanical nociception in conscious dogs. Vet Anaesth Analg 2016;43(2):215–26.
61. Giorgi M, Łebkowska-Wieruszewska B, Lisowski A, et al. Pharmacokinetic profiles of the active metamizole metabolites after four different routes of administration in healthy dogs. J Vet Pharmacol Ther 2018;41(3):428–36.
62. Zanuzzo FS, Teixeira-Neto FJ, Thomazini CM, et al. Effects of dipyrone, meloxicam, or the combination on hemostasis in conscious dogs. J Vet Emerg Crit Care 2015;25(4):512–20.
63. Lebkowska-Wieruszewska B, Kim TW, Chea B, et al. Pharmacokinetic profiles of the two major active metabolites of metamizole (dipyrone) in cats following three different routes of administration. J Vet Pharmacol Ther 2018;41(2):334–9.
64. Aharon MA, Prittie JE, Buriko K. A review of associated controversies surrounding glucocorticoid use in veterinary emergency and critical care. J Vet Emerg Crit Care 2017;27(3):267–77.

Alternatives to Opioid Analgesia in Small Animal Anesthesia: Alpha-2 Agonists

Alexander Valverde, DVM, DVSc[a],*,
Alicia M. Skelding, DVM, MSc, DVSc[b]

KEYWORDS

- Receptor • Xylazine • Medetomidine • Dexmedetomidine • Epidural • Intrathecal
- Constant rate infusion

KEY POINTS

- The sedation induced by alpha-2 agonists confounds the interpretation of analgesic effects but is also a part of the general analgesic effect that involves supraspinal and spinal mechanisms.
- Low systemic single doses can minimize sedative effects and provide analgesia, but it tends to be of short duration.
- Alternatively, specific administration of low doses at the site of action (eg, spinal cord) can provide analgesia of longer duration with minimal sedation.

INTRODUCTION

Alpha-2 agonists have desirable effects, including sedation, analgesia, and minimum alveolar concentration (MAC) sparing for inhalational anesthetics, and despite profound cardiovascular effects (hypertension/hypotension, bradycardia, and decreased cardiac output) they can also provide hemodynamic stability by controlling blood pressure.[1–12] The sedation induced by alpha-2 agonists confounds the interpretation of analgesic effects but is also a part of the general analgesic effect that involves supraspinal and spinal mechanisms. Low systemic single doses can minimize sedative effects and provide analgesia, but they tend to be of short duration. Alternatively, specific administration of low doses at the site of action (eg, spinal cord) can provide analgesia of longer duration with minimal sedation.

Disclosures: None.
[a] Department of Clinical Studies, Ontario Veterinary College, University of Guelph, Guelph, Ontario N1G 2W1, Canada; [b] Toronto Animal Health Partners Emergency and Specialty Hospital, Toronto, Ontario M3B 2R2, Canada
* Corresponding author.
E-mail address: valverde@uoguelph.ca

PAIN AND THE NORADRENERGIC ANTINOCICEPTIVE PATHWAY

Ascending pain transmission can be described in simple terms as a relay of nociceptive information via 3 steps: (1) the activation of peripheral nociceptive fibers (A-delta and C fibers; first-order neurons) by noxious stimulation and relay to laminae I and II in the dorsal horn of the spinal cord; (2) the activation of spinal tracts (second-order neurons) by neurotransmitters (eg, substance P and glutamate) released from first-order neurons that relay this information to the thalamus, which conveys this information also to the hypothalamus and amygdala, the periaqueductal gray, and the rostral ventromedial medulla (RVM); and (3) perception of pain once the cortex is stimulated by third-order neurons.[13,14]

The descending noradrenergic pathway is antinociceptive and originates from the locus coeruleus and the pontine region of the brain, and projects to the dorsal horn, where it inhibits pain signaling from the nociceptive A-delta and C fibers.[13–16] All these regions communicate with the periaqueductal gray and the RVM and are simultaneously activated when ascending pain transmission occurs, to constitute part of the endogenous pain inhibitory system, which also includes opioidergic, serotonergic, and dopaminergic systems.[13,14] These descending inhibitory pathways can interact and be synergistic at different levels of the pain pathway, and have a major role in modulating pain.[13–15]

ALPHA-ADRENERGIC DRUGS AND ANTINOCICEPTION

Alpha-2 agonists include xylazine, detomidine, romifidine, medetomidine, and dexmedetomidine. Dexmedetomidine is currently the most commonly used alpha-2 agonist in small animal practice and has replaced xylazine. Xylazine has been implicated as a risk factor for increased odds of death in studies from the 1990s,[17,18] but not medetomidine (equal mixture of dexmedetomidine and levomedetomidine) in more recent studies,[19] which may be the result of better alpha-2 to alpha-1 specificity, better understanding of pharmacodynamic properties of these drugs, and/or superior monitoring techniques nowadays.

Alpha-2 Adrenergic Receptors

Alpha-adrenergic receptors are G_i protein–coupled transmembrane receptors[20–22] that specifically inhibit adenylyl cyclase when stimulated, decreasing the synthesis of cyclic AMP, as well as activate G protein–coupled inward rectifying potassium channels.[5,16,21,22] These receptors are distributed throughout the peripheral and central nervous systems and other tissues.[5,15,21,23] Their wide distribution in the spinal cord and brain is responsible for their antinociceptive actions when stimulated by an alpha-2 adrenergic agonist.

Alpha-2 receptor subtypes include alpha-2a, alpha-2b, and alpha-2c, based on specific affinity for alpha adrenoceptor ligands, tissue location, and species in which they were identified, and all subtypes are involved in antinociceptive actions.[5,24,25]

All subtypes bind alpha-2 agonists and antagonists with similar affinities.[5,21] Alpha-2 receptors are located presynaptically (alpha-2a and alpha-2c) on the membrane of sympathetic nerve endings and inhibit the release of norepinephrine to modulate sympathetic effects.[5] All 3 receptor subtypes are also located postsynaptically in different tissues to exert various physiologic functions: alpha-2a receptors are located in the brain and spinal cord, where they mediate sedative, neuroprotective, antinociceptive, body temperature regulation, and sympatholytic effects[5,26–28]; peripherally, they also inhibit insulin secretion from pancreatic β cells and cause vasoconstriction of large arteries.[29,30] Alpha-2b receptors are located in the spinal cord and peripheral circulation and mediate antinociception and vasoconstriction in small arteries and veins, respectively.[5,28,29] Alpha-2c receptors are also present in the brain and spinal cord and mediate antinociception, cognition, behavior/mood, and locomotor inhibition, as well as peripherally for regulation of epinephrine outflow from the adrenal medulla and body temperature regulation.[5,25,28]

Alpha-adrenergic drugs can also interact with another class of receptor, the imidazoline receptor, in different regions of the brain.[20,31] The relevance of this receptor lies in its higher selectivity for alpha-2 than for alpha-1 adrenergic drugs, so that imidazole compounds (eg, dexmedetomidine) have a high affinity for both alpha-2 adrenergic and imidazoline receptors to which catecholamines (alpha-1 agonists) do not bind.[20] The interaction of alpha-2 agonists with the imidazoline-1 (I_1) receptor results in cardiovascular effects that are discussed later in this article, but are not linked to any analgesic effects.

Analgesic Site of Action

Alpha-2 agonists provide antinociception through supraspinal and spinal mechanisms. The sedative effects of these drugs (supraspinal effects) are the result of crossing the blood-brain barrier and suppressing noradrenergic neural activity at the locus coeruleus, which in turn can decrease pain perception, but it also causes direct antinociceptive effects through interference between second-order and third-order neurons and activation of descending inhibition noradrenergic pathways.[23,27]

The specific site of antinociceptive action of alpha-2 agonists at the level of the spinal cord is the dorsal gray matter (dorsal horn), where they selectively inhibit A-delta and C fiber–evoked activity in wide dynamic range neurons through presynaptic and postsynaptic actions.[15] Specifically, at the presynaptic level, alpha-2 agonists suppress the release of substance P and glutamate from afferent first-order neurons (A-delta and C fibers), which reduces excitatory postsynaptic potentials in second-order ascending neurons. Postsynaptically, alpha-2 agonists hyperpolarize second-order neurons in the substantia gelatinosa at the dorsal horn,[15,16] which enhances modulation and decreases projection of ascending nociceptive information.

Alpha-1 receptor agonistic actions could also result in analgesia but only at doses that result in hyperreflexia, which is related to actions on the ventral horn through facilitation of C fiber–evoked reflexes, and therefore they are not clinically useful.[15] Alpha-2 adrenergic agonists are able to suppress this ventral horn outflow and prevent motor excitability,[15] while still providing analgesia.

It has been shown that the mixed alpha-1 and alpha-2 agonistic effects can affect the analgesic actions of alpha-2 agonists. In mice, blockade of the alpha-1 receptor agonistic activity can restore and/or enhance the analgesic effects of the alpha-2 receptor agonistic activity.[32] Therefore, it is suggested that drugs with greater alpha-2 selectivity are preferred for analgesic actions.[32] Such drugs include dexmedetomidine, which has the highest alpha-2 to alpha-1 selectivity of all alpha-2 agonists at 1620, more than 160 for xylazine and 260 for detomidine[33]; however, the analgesic effects of different alpha-2 agonist drugs have not been compared to demonstrate this difference.

ANALGESIC CLINICAL USES

Alpha-2 agonists can provide analgesia through any of several routes of administration, including parenteral, oral, epidural, or intrathecal and intra-articular, because of spinal and supraspinal actions. The antinociceptive effects of dexmedetomidine were compared for several of these routes and found to have the best relative antinociceptive activity in this order: intrathecal > epidural ≥ parenteral, for skin twitch and paw pressure tests applied to the hind limb, but this antinociceptive activity was only evident in the forelimb and equivalent to hind limb for parenteral administration. The intrathecal and epidural catheters were positioned at L2-L3 spinal segments, relevant to hind limb innervation.[4]

Parenteral Analgesia

Both spinal and supraspinal actions contribute to the analgesic effects of alpha-2 agonists, and it seems that the sedative effects outlast the analgesic effects. Administration of 20 µg/kg, intravenous (IV) of medetomidine or 10 µg/kg, intramuscular (IM), of dexmedetomidine to conscious dogs resulted in sedation that outlasted the duration of analgesia, tested with toe-pinch stimulation,[6,10] but it is not clear whether analgesia is of less duration because sedation biases the interpretation of pain.[34]

Using pain models, alpha-2 agonists have been tested in conscious cats for thermal antinociception, and doses of 40 µg/kg, IM, of dexmedetomidine caused a significant increase in the nociceptive threshold for up to 3 hours; however, it was still inferior to buprenorphine.[35] Use of lower doses, 5 to 20 µg/kg, IV, of dexmedetomidine also resulted in significant analgesia but of shorter duration (45 minutes) using the same pain model.[34] Oral transmucosal (OTM) administration of 40 µg/kg of dexmedetomidine and using the same pain model resulted in a similar degree of analgesia and sedation to the same IM dose.[36] The physicochemical properties of dexmedetomidine, including a pKa of 7.1, lipophilic, and small molecular weight, and the oral pH of cats of 8 to 9, make the use of dexmedetomidine by OTM route ideal because of increased bioavailability.[36] In aggressive dogs, OTM dexmedetomidine has also been used at a dose of 33 µg/kg with satisfactory sedation, but analgesia was not assessed,[37] and a commercial formulation for OTM dexmedetomidine is now available and used for treatment of anxiety and noise aversion in dogs.[38]

In dogs under isoflurane anesthesia, nociceptive withdrawal reflex and temporal summation to repeated electrical stimulation of the lateral plantar digital nerve, to denote truly nociceptive effects, were determined after a bolus of 1 µg/kg, IV, of dexmedetomidine, followed by a continuous-rate infusion of 1 µg/kg/h, and showed suppression of nociceptive reflex responses that can prevent the development of postoperative chronic pain.[39]

Epidural Analgesia

Epidural administration of alpha-2 agonists allows diffusion across the dura and arachnoid mater to reach alpha-2 receptors in the superficial laminae of the dorsal horn to produce analgesia,[15] but they do not produce complete anesthesia because they do not affect all afferent or efferent fibers that constitute the spinal nerve. For example, intrathecal alpha-2 agonists have no effect on placing, stepping, or pinna twitch reflexes in rats, unless several times the antinociceptive dose is administered, which can result in hind limb flaccidity.[40] They can induce a differential nerve block in which C fibers are blocked to a greater extent than A-alpha fibers,[41] and their effects on A-delta fibers are also significant,[42] but in general they do not produce complete anesthesia or motor paralysis.[4]

Studies in horses have shown analgesia/anesthesia from epidural xylazine, similar to that of epidural lidocaine, to allow surgical procedures such as rectovaginal laceration repair, replacement of prolapsed rectum, and urethral extension,[43,44] but not from other alpha-2 agonists, and a local anesthetic effect from xylazine has been implicated.[45] However, dogs undergoing ovariohysterectomy with a combination of epidural lidocaine and xylazine had to be supplemented with isoflurane in some cases to complete the surgery, and similar results were obtained if the alpha-2 agonist was romifidine, dexmedetomidine, clonidine, or detomidine.[46]

When combined epidurally with opioids or local anesthetics, alpha-2 agonists can enhance the degree of analgesia and prolong the duration of action of other drugs, including local anesthetics, through synergistic interactions (**Table 1**).[15,47,48] In dogs undergoing pelvic limb orthopedic surgery, dexmedetomidine added to bupivacaine compared well for analgesia with morphine and bupivacaine, but resulted in longer time for return of pelvic limb motor function.[48] However, in dogs undergoing anesthesia for surgical correction of cranial cruciate ligament rupture, no major benefit in postoperative analgesia was obtained by adding epidural medetomidine to morphine, compared with epidural morphine alone.[49]

Systemic absorption of alpha-2 agonists from the epidural space is significant because the doses used epidurally are similar to systemic doses and the rate of absorption is similar to that of an IM injection; therefore, analgesia can be the result of spinal and supraspinal actions. Systemic absorption also results in the characteristic effects of these drugs on the cardiorespiratory system, in addition to sedation and adverse effects, discussed later in relation to systemic effects.

Intrathecal Analgesia

Intrathecal (subarachnoid or spinal) injection usually requires reduced doses because the drug is deposited in close proximity to the site of action (spinal cord) and has already bypassed the barrier of the dura and arachnoid mater. The systemic effects are less likely because the low doses administered intrathecally also result in very slow absorption into the circulation, and therefore the analgesia that results is more likely to be from a spinal action only.

Intrathecal administration of alpha-2 agonists does not result in the biphasic blood pressure response, typical of systemic administration, but results in immediate blockade of sympathetic outflow that results in persistent bradycardia and hypotension. In sheep, intrathecal dexmedetomidine resulted in a larger and more rapid decrease in arterial blood pressure within 2 minutes of injection than epidural administration.[50]

The use of intrathecal alpha-2 agonists has not been thoroughly evaluated in dogs and cats. In dogs, intrathecal administration of dexmedetomidine (0.66 μg/kg) resulted in greater antinociceptive effects than epidural administration (3.33 μg/kg) to prevent skin twitch or paw withdrawal of the hind limb.[4] The ED_{50} (50% effective dose) to achieve those effects with intrathecal administration was 20% to 25% of the epidural dose.[4]

Intraarticular

The intraarticular route has been reported in human anesthesia with dexmedetomidine, in patients undergoing surgical procedures of the knee, such as partial meniscectomy, diagnostic arthroscopy, and reconstruction of the cruciate ligaments.[51,52] In these studies, a dose of 1 μg/kg of dexmedetomidine was mixed in 20 mL of saline and injected in patients under general inhalant anesthesia[51] or doses of 1 or 2 μg/kg of dexmedetomidine mixed with 18 mL of ropivacaine, injected in patients under spinal anesthesia into the joint postsurgery,[52] before removal of the tourniquet applied for surgery and until 10 minutes after the intraarticular injection. In both studies, the visual analog pain scores were significantly lower with the addition of dexmedetomidine compared with control groups of saline or IV dexmedetomidine (1 μg/kg)[51] or intraarticular ropivacaine alone.[52] This information denotes a local effect, because intraarticular dexmedetomidine was superior to IV

Table 1
Alpha-2 agonists administered epidurally at the lumbosacral space and associated duration of analgesia

Alpha-2 Agonist (Dose)	Other Epidural Analgesic (1 mg/kg)	Duration of Analgesia (h)	Method to Assess Analgesia	Reference
Dog				
Medetomidine (5 μg/kg)	Morphine (0.11)	13.1 ± 3.1	Towel clamp applied to the tail	Branson et al,[47] 1993
Medetomidine (5 μg/kg)	None	No analgesia	Towel clamp applied to the tail	Branson et al,[47] 1993
Medetomidine (15 μg/kg)	None	7.1 ± 0.5	Postoperative pain after orthopedic surgery of the pelvis or hind limb	Vesal et al,[83] 1996
Dexmedetomidine (4 μg/kg)	Bupivacaine (1)	No postoperative rescue analgesia required for 24	Postoperative pain after pelvic limb orthopedic surgery	O & Smith,[48] 2013
Dexmedetomidine (2 μg/kg)	Lidocaine with epinephrine (2.5)	Up to 3	Ovariohysterectomy	Pohl et al,[46] 2012
Dexmedetomidine (1.5, 3, 6 μg/kg)	None	Not determined	Isoflurane MAC reduction by 13 ± 10%, 29 ± 5%, and 31 ± 6%; respectively	Campagnol et al,[84] 2007
Xylazine (0.25 mg/kg)	Lidocaine with epinephrine (2.5)	Up to 4	Ovariohysterectomy	Pohl et al,[46] 2012
Xylazine (0.1, 0.2, 0.4 mg/kg)	None	Not determined	Isoflurane MAC reduction by 8 ± 3%, 22 ± 5%, and 33 ± 3%, respectively	Soares et al,[85] 2004
Detomidine (30 μg/kg)	Lidocaine with epinephrine (2.5)	Up to 3	Ovariohysterectomy	Pohl et al,[46] 2012
Romifidine (10 μg/kg)	Lidocaine with epinephrine (2.5)	Up to 3	Ovariohysterectomy	Pohl et al,[46] 2012
Clonidine (5 μg/kg)	Lidocaine with epinephrine (2.5)	Up to 3	Ovariohysterectomy	Pohl et al,[46] 2012
Cat				
Medetomidine (10 μg/kg)	None	4 for the pelvic limb 2 for the thoracic limb	Electrical cutaneous stimulus	Duke et al,[73] 1994
Dexmedetomidine (4 μg/kg)	Lidocaine (1)	Intraoperatively	Ovariohysterectomy; lower isoflurane requirements than for cats receiving epidural lidocaine alone	Souza et al,[86] 2010

dexmedetomidine,[51] and involves alpha-2 presynaptic receptors and actions on C and A-delta fibers.[41,53]

The adverse effects of alpha-2a receptor activation in the joint should be considered, because clonidine has been shown to intensify cartilage degradation and subchondral bone deterioration in rats with induced osteoarthritis of the temporomandibular joint,[54] which may involve a pro-osteoclastic effect of alpha-2a signaling via promotion of osteoclast maturation and induction of apoptosis of articular chondrocytes.[55]

Adjunct to Local Anesthetics

The addition of alpha-2 agonists to local anesthetics for peripheral nerve blocks has been found to prolong the duration of action of the local anesthetic through actions on the peripheral alpha-2a receptor.[56] The proposed mechanism of action is by prolonging the hyperpolarization of the nerve fiber via inhibition of the hyperpolarization cation current,[57,58] and to some extent by vasoconstriction induced by the alpha-2 agonist, which may delay the systemic absorption of the local anesthetic agent in a similar manner to the addition of epinephrine, thereby prolonging its peripheral effect.[56]

Studies in dogs and cats have not been conclusive. Addition of dexmedetomidine (1 μg/mL) to ropivacaine 0.75% for sciatic and femoral nerve blockade in dogs showed some prolongation in the duration of sensory block, but not for motor blockade.[59] The addition of medetomidine (10 μg/kg) to mepivacaine (5 mg/kg) or administration of medetomidine (10 μg/kg, IM) with local infiltration of mepivacaine for peripheral radial nerve block prolonged sensory and motor blockade compared with the same dose of mepivacaine alone[60]; however, the effects of medetomidine could have resulted from systemic effects.

In cats, the addition of dexmedetomidine (1 μg/kg) to bupivacaine (0.46 mg/kg) for femoral and sciatic nerve blockade showed no benefits compared with the use of the same dose of bupivacaine alone for peripheral nerve block and analgesia.[61]

SYSTEMIC EFFECTS

Alpha-2 agonists can elicit multiple systemic effects that should be considered when administered for analgesic purposes. The following systemic effects are the most relevant.

Sedation

Sedative effects of alpha-2 agonists are related to alpha-2 receptor interactions, most likely related to the alpha-2a receptors, located in neurons of the locus coeruleus.[5,62] Alpha-2 agonists are potent sedatives, but their combination with opioids also results in longer sedation and better analgesia than the alpha-2 agonist alone,[6,10] because of synergistic actions.[15]

Minimum Alveolar Concentration Sparing

The effects of alpha-2 agonists on decreasing the MAC of inhalational anesthetics have been shown in several studies. These effects are also related to interactions with alpha-2a receptors, both supraspinal and spinal.[3,62,63] The MAC-sparing effect can result from parenteral or epidural/intrathecal administration (see **Table 1**; **Table 2**), and administration of the antagonist atipamezole can completely reverse the MAC-sparing effect of parenterally administered alpha-2 agonists.[64,65] The effect of atipamezole on epidural/intrathecal alpha-2 agonists and MAC has not been investigated. Interestingly, atipamezole alone does not affect the MAC of isoflurane.[65]

Activation of imidazoline receptors has no effect on MAC.[63]

Table 2
Effects of alpha-2 agonists on the minimum alveolar concentrations of inhalants

Alpha-2 Agonist (Dose; Route)	Species	Inhalant MAC Reduction (%)	Reference
Medetomidine (30 µg/kg; IV)	Canine	Isoflurane 47	Ewing et al,[65] 1993
Medetomidine (2 µg/kg; IV) Followed by 0.5 and 1.0 µg/kg/h, IV	Canine	Desflurane 11–15[a]	Gómez-Villamondos et al,[87] 2008
Dexmedetomidine (20 µg/kg, IV)	Canine	Isoflurane 86	Weitz et al,[64] 1991
Dexmedetomidine (3 µg/kg, IV)	Canine	Isoflurane 71	Nguyen et al,[72] 1992
Dexmedetomidine (0.1 µg/kg/h, IV) (0.5 µg/kg/h, IV) (3 µg/kg/h, IV)	Canine	Isoflurane 6 18 59	Pascoe et al,[88] 2006
Dexmedetomidine (0.5 µg/kg/h, IV)	Canine	Isoflurane 30	Ebner et al,[9] 2013
Dexmedetomidine (1.5 µg/kg, IV) Followed by 1.5 µg/kg/h, IV (4.5 µg/kg, IV) Followed by 4.5 µg/kg/h, IV	Canine	Sevoflurane 44 69	Hector et al,[81] 2017
Dexmedetomidine Plasma concentrations of 0.08–25.21 ng/mL	Feline	Isoflurane up to 77 at the highest plasma concentration	Pypendop et al,[82] 2019
Dexmedetomidine Plasma concentrations of 0.06–11.46 ng/mL	Feline	Isoflurane up to 77 at the highest plasma concentration	Escobar et al,[89] 2012

[a] Assessed as prevention of movement to tail clamping during anesthesia.

Cardiorespiratory

The use of alpha-2 adrenergic agonists as sole analgesic drugs is limited by their strong sedative effects and profound cardiovascular depression. The cardiovascular effects elicited by alpha-2 adrenergic drugs have been associated with actions on both the adrenergic and imidazoline receptors. The vasoconstrictor effects of alpha-2 agonists are specifically mediated through postsynaptic alpha-1 and alpha-2 (predominantly alpha-2b) receptor actions,[29] which result in an increase in vascular resistance/hypertension and reflex bradycardia.[1] Presynaptic effects of alpha-2a and alpha-2c receptors act as autoreceptors by inhibiting the release of their own neurotransmitter, norepinephrine, from sympathetic nerve endings and central adrenergic neurons,[5] an important effect for blood pressure regulation. The actions on both presynaptic and postsynaptic receptors is responsible for the biphasic blood pressure response seen with alpha-2 agonists, of initial hypertension from postsynaptic actions, followed by hypotension from presynaptic actions.[5,65]

The actions on the imidazoline receptor can be cardiovascular protective, specifically through the I_1 receptor.[21,31,66] For example, dexmedetomidine can prevent epinephrine-induced arrhythmias in halothane-anesthetized dogs through its actions on the imidazoline receptor.[67] Similarly, the antihypertensive effects of drugs such as clonidine (imidazoline compound), also an agonist on the alpha-2 adrenergic and imidazoline receptor, are also mediated through the imidazoline receptor.[20]

Typical cardiovascular effects from alpha-2 agonists administered to conscious dogs include an increase in vascular resistance, which results in hypertension, reflex bradycardia with atrioventricular blocks, and sinus arrhythmia, and sometimes escape beats, reductions in cardiac output, increases in central venous pressure, and hypotension over time.[6,10,68]

The concurrent administration of inhalant anesthetics ameliorate some of these effects because of the vasodilatory effects of the inhalant, especially with regard to heart rate, rhythm, and hypertension.[8,9,11,12,68] In both scenarios, there are decreases in oxygen delivery and the extraction ratio of oxygen, but organ perfusion and oxygenation remain within acceptable levels.[9,12,68–70]

The respiratory effects of alpha-2 agonists involve a significant decrease in respiratory rate from sedative effects, without concurrent significant changes in $Paco_2$ and Pao_2, whether administered to conscious or anesthetized patients.[6,8,10,11] Doses as low as 5 µg/kg of medetomidine can cause respiratory depression in isoflurane-anesthetized dogs through decreases in rate and tidal volume, because of decreased respiratory center output.[71] Because of significant reduction in inhalant requirements (MAC sparing) induced by alpha-2 agonists, the adjustment in end-tidal concentrations of the inhalant can maintain relatively normal respiratory function and minimize respiratory depression compared with the effects seen with inhalant anesthesia alone.[72]

Vomiting

Vomiting seems to be more common in cats than in dogs. More than 75% of conscious cats vomited within 6.4 minutes of epidural medetomidine administration[73] and within 10 minutes of IM or OTM dexmedetomidine administration.[36]

Pupillary Size

In cats and rats, alpha-2 agonists have been reported to induce pupillary dilation (mydriasis) by a central postsynaptic effect through stimulation of ascending inhibitory mechanisms that result in norepinephrine release and activation of inhibitory alpha-2 receptors on the neurons of the Edinger-Westphal complex, where preganglionic parasympathetic fibers to the iris originate and cause pupillary constriction.[1,74] In contrast, in dogs and people, the effect is pupillary constriction (miosis) in dogs[75,76] or no change in pupil size in people,[77] and the effects have been related to sympathetic inhibition or actions on alpha-2 receptors close to or in the pupilloconstrictor nucleus that produce miosis and also reduce reflex dilation of the pupil.[77]

ANTAGONISTS

Alpha-2 antagonists include drugs with central/peripheral antagonistic actions, such as atipamezole,[65] and drugs with only peripheral antagonistic actions, such as vatinoxan (previously known as L-659,066 or MK 0467).[78–80]

A central/peripheral antagonist can reverse all effects of alpha-2 agonists, including analgesia. Doses of 50 µg/kg of atipamezole, IM, can reverse sedation induced by 5 µg/kg, IV, of dexmedetomidine,[78] and doses of 0.3 mg/kg, IV, can completely reverse the sparing effect of medetomidine on isoflurane MAC, whereas administration of atipamezole alone does not have any effect on MAC.[65]

Vatinoxan has been shown to attenuate the cardiovascular effects of dexmedetomidine that result from the increase in vascular resistance, without affecting sedation.[78–80] Vatinoxan administration without concurrent use of dexmedetomidine has been shown to increase the MAC of sevoflurane in dogs by 10% to 19%[81] and the MAC of isoflurane by 21% in cats[82]; in addition, it lessened the maximum MAC reduction of isoflurane induced by dexmedetomidine in cats by 22%.[82]

However, the effects of these antagonists on analgesia have not been determined in dose-titrated studies.

REFERENCES

1. Virtanen R, MacDonald E. Comparison of the effects of detomidine and xylazine on some alpha 2-adrenoceptor-mediated responses in the central and peripheral nervous systems. Eur J Pharmacol 1985;115(2–3):277–84.

2. Pypendop BH, Verstegen JP. Hemodynamic effects of medetomidine in the dog: a dose titration study. Vet Surg 1998;27(6):612–22.

3. Segal IS, Vickery RG, Walton JK, et al. Dexmedetomidine diminishes halothane anesthetic requirements in rats through a postsynaptic alpha2-adrenergic receptor. Anesthesiology 1988;69(6):818–23.

4. Sabbe MB, Penning JP, Ozaki GT, et al. Spinal and systemic action of the α2 receptor agonist dexmedetomidine in dogs. Anesthesiology 1994;80(5):1057–72.

5. Philipp M, Brede M, Hein L. Physiological significance of $α_2$-adrenergic receptor subtype diversity: one receptor is not enough. Am J Physiol Regul Integr Comp Physiol 2002;283(2):R287–95.

6. Kuo WC, Keegan RD. Comparative cardiovascular, analgesic, and sedative effects of medetomidine, medetomidine-hydromorphone, and medetomidine-butorphanol in dogs. Am J Vet Res 2004;65(7):931–7.

7. Murrell JC, Hellebrekers LJ. Medetomidine and dexmedetomidine: a review of cardiovascular effects and antinociceptive properties in the dog. Vet Anaesth Analg 2005;32(3):17–27.

8. Congdon JM, Marquez M, Niyom S, et al. Cardiovascular, respiratory, electrolyte and acid-base balance during continuous dexmedetomidine infusion in anesthetized dogs. Vet Anaesth Analg 2013;40(5):464–71.

9. Ebner LS, Lerche P, Bednarski RM, et al. Effect of dexmedetomidine, morphine-lidocaine-ketamine, and dexmedetomidine-morphine-lidocaine-ketamine constant rate infusions on the minimum alveolar concentration of isoflurane and bispectral index in dogs. Am J Vet Res 2013;74(7):963–70.

10. Cardoso CG, Marques DRC, da Silva THM, et al. Cardiorespiratory, sedative and antinociceptive effects of dexmedetomidine alone or in combination with methadone, morphine or tramadol in dogs. Vet Anaesth Analg 2014;41(6):636–43.

11. Pascoe PJ. The cardiopulmonary effects of dexmedetomidine infusions in dogs during isoflurane anesthesia. Vet Anaesth Analg 2015;42(4):360–8.

12. Moran-Muñoz R, Valverde A, Ibancovichi JA, et al. Cardiovascular effects of constant rate infusions of lidocaine, lidocaine and dexmedetomidine, and dexmedetomidine in dogs anesthetized at equipotent doses of sevoflurane. Can Vet J 2017;58(7):729–34.

13. Ossipov MH, Dussor GO, Porreca F. Central modulation of pain. J Clin Invest 2010;120(11):3779–87.

14. Kwon M, Altin M, Duenas H, et al. The role of descending inhibitory pathways on chronic pain modulation and clinical implications. Pain Pract 2013;14(7):656–67.

15. Yaksh TL. Pharmacology of spinal adrenergic systems which modulate spinal nociceptive processing. Pharmacol Biochem Behav 1985;22(5):845–58.

16. Sonohata M, Furue H, Katafuchi T, et al. Actions of noradrenaline on substantia gelatinosa neurones in the rat spinal cord revealed by *in vivo* patch recording. J Physiol 2004;555(Pt 2):515–26.

17. Dyson DH, Maxie MG, Schnurr D. Morbidity and mortality associated with anesthetic management in small animal veterinary practice in Ontario. J Am Anim Hosp Assoc 1998;34(4):325–35.

18. Clarke KW, Hall LW. A survey of anaesthesia in small animal practice: AVA/BSAVA report. J Ass Vet Anaesth 1990;17(1):4–10.

19. Brodbelt D. Perioperative mortality in small animal anaesthesia. Vet J 2009; 182(2):152–61.

20. Codd EE, Press JB, Raffa RB. Alpha$_2$-adrenoceptors vs. imidazoline receptors: implications for α_2-mediated analgesia and other non-cardiovascular therapeutic uses. Life Sci 1995;56(2):63–74.

21. Khan ZP, Ferguson CN, Jones RM. Alpha-2 and imidazoline receptor agonists. Their pharmacology and therapeutic role. Anaesthesia 1999;54(2):146–65.

22. Pierce KL, Premont RT, Lefkowitz RJ. Seven-transmembrane receptors. Nat Rev Mol Cell Biol 2002;3(9):639–50.

23. Schmitt H, Le Douarec JC, Petillot N. Antinociceptive effects of some α-sympathomimetic agents. Neuropharmacology 1974;13(5):289–94.

24. Stone LS, MacMillan LB, Kitto KF, et al. The α_{2a} adrenergic receptor subtype mediates spinal analgesia evoked by α_2 agonists and is necessary for spinal adrenergic-opioid synergy. J Neurosci 1997;17(18):7157–65.

25. Fairbanks CA, Stone LS, Kitto KF, et al. α_{2c}-adrenergic receptors mediate spinal analgesia and adrenergic-opioid synergy. J Pharmacol Exp Ther 2002;300(1): 282–90.

26. Ma D, Hossain M, Rajakumaraswamy N, et al. Dexmedetomidine produces it neuroprotective effect via the alpha 2A-adrenoceptor subtype. Eur J Pharmacol 2004;502(1–2):87–97.

27. Zhang Z, Ferretti V, Güntan I, et al. Neuronal ensembles sufficient for recovery sleep and the sedative actions of α_2 adrenergic agonists. Nat Neurosci 2015; 18(4):553–61.

28. Giovannitti JA, Thoms SM, Crawford JJ. Alpha-2 adrenergic receptor agonists: a review of current clinical applications. Anesth Prog 2015;62(1):31–8.

29. Kanagy NL. α_2-adrenergic receptor signalling in hypertension. Clin Sci 2005; 109(5):431–7.

30. Fagerholm V, Scheinin M, Haaparanta M. Alpha2A-adrenoceptor antagonism increases insulin secretion and synergistically augments the insulinotropic effect of glibenclamide in mice. Br J Pharmacol 2008;154(6):1287–96.

31. Ernsberger P, Friedman JE, Koletsky RJ. The I$_1$-imidazoline receptor: from binding site to therapeutic target in cardiovascular disease. J Hypertens Suppl 1997; 15(1):S9–23.

32. Gil DW, Cheevers CV, Kedzie KM, et al. α-1 adrenergic receptor agonist activity of clinical α-adrenergic receptor agonists interferes with α-2 mediated analgesia. Anesthesiology 2009;110(2):401–7.

33. Virtanen R, Savola JM, Saano V, et al. Characterization of the selectivity, specificity and potency of medetomidine as an α_2-adrenoceptor agonist. Eur J Pharmacol 1988;150(1–2):9–14.

34. Pypendop BH, Ilkiw JE. Relationship between plasma dexmedetomidine concentration and sedation score and thermal threshold in cats. Am J Vet Res 2014; 75(5):446–52.

35. Slingsby LS, Taylor PM. Thermal antinociception after dexmedetomidine administration in cats: a dose-finding study. J Vet Pharmacol Ther 2008;31(2):135–42.

36. Slingsby LS, Taylor PM, Monroe T. Thermal antinociception after dexmedetomidine administration in cats: a comparison between intramuscular and oral transmucosal administration. J Feline Med Surg 2009;11(10):829–34.

37. Cohen AE, Bennett SL. Oral transmucosal administration of dexmedetomidine for sedation in 4 dogs. Can Vet J 2015;56(11):1144–8.

38. Korpivaara M, Laapas K, Huhtinen M, et al. Dexmedetomidine oromucosal gel for noise-associated acute anxiety and fear in dogs- a randomised, double-blind, placebo-controlled clinical study. Vet Rec 2017;180(14):356–62.

39. Lervik A, Haga HA, Ranheim B, et al. The influence of a continuous rate infusion of dexmedetomidine on the nociceptive withdrawal reflex and temporal summation during isoflurane anaesthesia in dogs. Vet Anaesth Analg 2012;39(4):414–25.

40. Reddy SVR, Maderdrut JL, Yaksh TL. Spinal cord pharmacology of adrenergic agonist-mediated antinociception. J Pharmacol Exp Ther 1980;213(3):525–33.

41. Butterworth JF, Strichartz GR. The α_2-adrenergic agonists clonidine and guanfacine produce tonic and phasic block of conduction in rat sciatic nerve fibers. Anesth Analg 1993;76(2):295–301.

42. Kawasaki Y, Kumamoto E, Furue H, et al. α^2 adrenoceptor-mediated presynaptic inhibition of primary afferent glutamatergic transmission in rat substantia gelatinosa neurons. Anesthesiology 2003;98(3):682–9.

43. Fikes LW, Lin HC, Thurmon JC. A preliminary comparison of lidocaine and xylazine as epidural analgesics in ponies. Vet Surg 1989;18(1):85–6.

44. LeBlanc PH, Caron JP. Clinical use of epidural xylazine in the horse. Equine Vet J 1990;22(3):180–1.

45. Aziz MA, Martin RJ. α agonist and local anaesthetic properties of xylazine. Zentralbl Veterinarmed A 1978;25(3):181–8.

46. Pohl VH, Carregaro AB, Lopes C, et al. Epidural anesthesia and postoperatory analgesia with alpha-2 adrenergic agonists and lidocaine for ovariohysterectomy in bitches. Can J Vet Res 2012;76(3):215–20.

47. Branson KR, Ko JCH, Tranquilli WJ, et al. Duration of analgesia induced by epidurally administered morphine and medetomidine in dogs. J Vet Pharmacol Ther 1993;16(3):369–72.

48. O O, Smith LJ. A comparison of epidural analgesia provided by bupivacaine alone, bupivacaine + morphine, or bupivacaine + dexmedetomidine for pelvic orthopedic surgery in dogs. Vet Anaesth Analg 2013;40(5):527–36.

49. Pacharinsak C, Greene SA, Keegan RD, et al. Postoperative analgesia in dogs receiving epidural morphine plus medetomidine. J Vet Pharmacol Ther 2003; 26(1):71–7.

50. Eisenach JC, Shafer SL, Bucklin BA, et al. Pharmacokinetics and pharmacodynamics of intraspinal dexmedetomidine in sheep. Anesthesiology 1994;80(6): 1349–59.

51. Al-Metwalli RR, Mowafi HA, Ismail SA, et al. Effect of intra-articular dexmedetomidine on postoperative analgesia after arthroscopic knee surgery. Br J Anaesth 2008;101(3):395–9.

52. Panigrahi R, Roy R, Mahapatra AK, et al. Intra-articular adjuvant analgesics following knee arthroscopy: comparison between single and double dose

dexmedetomidine and ropivacaine. A multicenter prospective double-blind trial. Orthop Surg 2015;7(3):250–5.

53. Gentili M, Juhel A, Bonnet F. Peripheral analgesic effect of intra-articular clonidine. Pain 1996;64(3):593–6.

54. Jiao K, Zeng G, Niu LN, et al. Activation of α-2A-adrenergic signal transduction in chondrocytes promotes degenerative remodelling of temporomandibular joint. Sci Rep 2016;6(1):30085.

55. Lorenz J, Schäfer N, Bauer R, et al. Norepinephrine modulates osteoarthritic chondrocyte metabolism and inflammatory responses. Osteoarthritis Cartilage 2016;24(2):325–34.

56. Yoshitomi Y, Kohjitani A, Maeda S, et al. Dexmedetomidine enhances the local anesthetic action of lidocaine via an α-2A adrenoceptor. Anesth Analg 2008; 107(1):96–101.

57. Brummett CM, Hong EK, Janda AM, et al. Perineural dexmedetomidine added to ropivacaine for sciatic nerve block in rats prolongs the duration of analgesia by blocking the hyperpolarization activated cation current. Anesthesiology 2011; 115(4):836–43.

58. Kirksey MA, Haskins SC, Cheng J, et al. Local anesthetic peripheral nerve block adjuvants for prolongation of analgesia: a systemic qualitative review. PLoS One 2015;10(9):e0137312.

59. Trein TA, Floriano BP, Waqatsuma JT, et al. Effects of dexmedetomidine combined with ropivacaine on sciatic and femoral nerve blockade in dogs. Vet Anaesth Analg 2017;44(1):144–53.

60. Lamont LA, Lemke KA. The effects of medetomidine on radial nerve blockade with mepivacaine in dogs. Vet Anaesth Analg 2008;35(1):62–8.

61. Evangelista MC, Doodnaught GM, Fantoni DT, et al. Sciatic and femoral nerve blockade using bupivacaine alone, or in combination with dexmedetomidine or buprenorphine in cats. Vet Rec 2017;180(24):592–7.

62. Lakhlani PP, MacMillan LB, Guo TZ, et al. Substitution of a mutant α_{2a}-adrenergic receptor via "hit and run" gene targeting reveals the role of this subtype in sedative, analgesic, and anesthetic sparing responses in vivo. Proc Natl Acad Sci U S A 1997;94(18):9950–5.

63. Kagawa K, Mammoto T, Hayashi Y, et al. The effect of imidazoline receptors and α_2-adrenoceptors on the anesthetic requirement (MAC) for halothane in rats. Anesthesiology 1997;87(4):963–7.

64. Weitz JD, Foster SD, Waugaman WR, et al. Anesthetic and hemodynamic effects of dexmedetomidine during isoflurane anesthesia in a canine model. Nurse Anesth 1991;2(1):19–27.

65. Ewing KIK, Mohammed HO, Scarlett JM, et al. Reduction of isoflurane anesthetic requirement by medetomidine and its restoration by atipamezole in dogs. Am J Vet Res 1993;54(2):294–9.

66. Li J-X, Zhang Y. Imidazoline I_2 receptors: target for new analgesics? Eur J Pharmacol 2011;658(2–3):49–56.

67. Kamibayashi T, Mammoto T, Hayashi Y, et al. Further characterization of the receptor mechanism involved in the antidysrhythmic effect of dexmedetomidine on halothane/epinephrine dysrhythmias in dogs. Anesthesiology 1995;83(5): 1082–9.

68. Pypendop BH, Barter LS, Stanley SD, et al. Hemodynamic effects of dexmedetomidine in isoflurane-anesthetized cats. Vet Anaesth Analg 2011;38(6):555–67.

69. Lawrence CJ, Prinzen FW, de Lange S. The effect of dexmedetomidine on nutrient organ blood flow. Anesth Analg 1996;83(6):1160–5.

70. Rioja E, Gianotti G, Valverde A. Clinical use of a low-dose medetomidine infusion in healthy dogs undergoing ovariohysterectomy. Can Vet J 2013;54(9):864–8.

71. Lerche P, Muir WW III. Effect of medetomidine on respiration and minimum alveolar concentration in halothane- and isoflurane-anesthetized dogs. Am J Vet Res 2006;67(5):782–9.

72. Nguyen D, Abdul-Rasool I, Ward D, et al. Ventilatory effects of dexmedetomidine, atipamezole, and isoflurane in dogs. Anesthesiology 1992;76:573–9.

73. Duke T, Cox AMK, Remedios AM, et al. The analgesic effects of administering fentanyl or medetomidine in the lumbosacral epidural space of cats. Vet Surg 1994;23(2):143–8.

74. Koss MC, Gherezeghiher T, Nomura A. CNS adrenergic inhibition of parasympathetic oculomotor tone. J Auton Nerv Syst 1984;10(1):55–68.

75. Artigas C, Redondo JI, López-Murcia MM. Effects of intravenous administration of dexmedetomidine on intraocular pressure and pupil size in clinically normal dogs. Vet Ophthalmol 2012;15(Suppl 1):79–82.

76. Micieli F, Chiavaccini L, Lamagna B, et al. Comparison of intraocular pressure and pupil diameter after sedation with either acepromazine or dexmedetomidine in healthy dogs. Vet Anaesth Analg 2018;45(5):667–72.

77. Larson MD, Talke PO. Effect of dexmedetomidine, an α_2-adrenoceptor agonist, on human pupillary reflexes during general anaesthesia. Br J Clin Pharmacol 2001;51(1):27–33.

78. Honkavaara JM, Raekallio MR, Juusela EK, et al. The effects of L-659,066, a peripheral α2-adrenoceptor antagonist, on dexmedetomidine-induced sedation and bradycardia in dogs. Vet Anaesth Analg 2008;35(5):409–13.

79. Enouri SS, Kerr CL, McDonell WN, et al. Effects of a peripheral alpha-2 adrenergic-receptor antagonist on the hemodynamic changes induced by medetomidine administration in conscious dogs. Am J Vet Res 2008;69(6):728–36.

80. Rolfe NG, Kerr CL, McDonell WN. Cardiopulmonary and sedative effects of the peripheral α2-adrenoceptor antagonist MK 0467 administered intravenously or intramuscularly concurrently with medetomidine in dogs. Am J Vet Res 2012; 73(5):587–94.

81. Hector RC, Rezende ML, Mama KR, et al. Effects of constant rate infusions of dexmedetomidine or MK-467 on the minimum alveolar concentration of sevoflurane in dogs. Vet Anaesth Analg 2017;44(4):755–65.

82. Pypendop BH, Ahokoivu H, Honkavaara J. Effects of dexmedetomidine, with or without vatinoxan (MK-467), on minimum alveolar concentration of isoflurane in cats. Vet Anaesth Analg 2019;46(4):443–51.

83. Vesal N, Cribb PH, Frketic M. Postoperative analgesic and cardiopulmonary effects in dogs of oxymorphone administered epidurally and intramuscularly, and medetomidine administered epidurally: a comparative clinical study. Vet Surg 1996;25(4):361–9.

84. Campagnol D, Teixeira Neto FJ, Giordano T, et al. Effects of epidural administration of dexmedetomidine on the minimum alveolar concentration of isoflurane in dogs. Am J Vet Res 2007;68(12):1308–18.

85. Soares JHN, Ascoli FO, Gremiao IDF, et al. Isoflurane sparing action of epidurally administered xylazine hydrochloride in anesthetized dogs. Am J Vet Res 2004; 65(6):854–9.

86. Souza SS, Intelisano TR, De Biaggi CP, et al. Cardiopulmonary and isoflurane-sparing effects of epidural or intravenous infusion of dexmedetomidine in cats undergoing surgery with epidural lidocaine. Vet Anaesth Analg 2010;37(2):106–15.

87. Gómez-Villamondos RJ, Palacios C, Benítez A, et al. Effect of medetomidine infusion on the anaesthetic requirements of desflurane in dogs. Res Vet Sci 2008; 84(1):68–73.

88. Pascoe PJ, Raekallio M, Kuusela E, et al. Changes in the minimum alveolar concentration of isoflurane and some cardiopulmonary measurements during three continuous infusion rates of dexmedetomidine in dogs. Vet Anaesth Analg 2006;33(2):97–103.

89. Escobar A, Pypendop BH, Siao KT, et al. Effect of dexmedetomidine on the minimum alveolar concentration of isoflurane in cats. J Vet Pharmacol Ther 2012; 35(2):163–8.

Acupuncture for the Treatment of Animal Pain

Bonnie D. Wright, DVM*

KEYWORDS

- Acupuncture • Neurophysiology • Fascia • Neuromodulation
- Mechanotransduction

KEY POINTS

- Acupuncture points are anatomically defined areas of the body that include myelinated and unmyelinated nerve fibers, low-threshold mechanoreceptors, mast cells, and microcirculatory complexes. This conglomerate is commonly referred to as the neural acupuncture unit.
- With needle placement, nerve stimulation occurs directly, or secondary to mechanical forces applied by the fascia in the region surrounding the acupuncture point.
- Acupuncture alters homeostasis via sympathetic/parasympathetic input, modification of axonal flow and dorsal root ganglion transcription, spinal neurotransmitter modulation, modification of reflex arcs, and influences on immune function.
- Central nervous system modification occurs in the form of stress reduction achieved by an increase in analgesic and inhibitory neurotransmitters from the periaqueductal gray and rostroventral medulla (regions of the brain that modulate pain pathways). This also contributes to increased activity of descending pain pathways and improved enteric homeostasis.
- Acupuncture has been shown to provide analgesia, reduce chronic pain, reduce addiction, and improve outcomes when used in addition to, or in place of, opioids.

INTRODUCTION

With the multifaceted regulatory issues surrounding opioids (opioid epidemic, availability issues, and increased regulation incentivizing abusers to pursue veterinary sources) as well as the ugly underbelly of opioid agonists being increasingly revealed (opioid-induced hyperalgesia, very poor absorption and utility of oral opioids in dogs, opioid-induced immune suppression, and the neuroinflammatory effects of opioids), nonopioid options for treating pain has become increasingly desirable.[1–3] In an

---

Disclosure Statement: Dr B.D. Wright teaches veterinary acupuncture courses through the canine rehabilitation institute. Her courses are supported, in part, by Lhasa Oms.
Colorado Canine Orthopedics and Rehabilitation
* 5520 N Nevada Ave #150, Colorado Springs, CO 80918.
E-mail address: mistralvet@gmail.com

attempt to stem the tide of addiction and address the emerging controversies surrounding opioids, regulatory agencies are recommending evidence-based treatments that are nonpharmacologic.[4] At the forefront of these techniques, especially where pain is concerned, is acupuncture,[5] a modality with deep roots and strong potential but plagued with equally deep misconceptions and consequent controversy.

Acupuncture consists of the stimulation of distinct anatomic points with fine needles. Other methods of stimulation of these points (such as injections, laser, deep pressure massage, trigger point needling) exist and are encompassed in the overall field of acupuncture-related modalities. The key differentiation between acupuncture with needles and other treatments is the source of force applied to the region of the acupuncture point. Other common sources of stimulation of acupuncture points are thermal, electrical, chemical, photons, and more.

The practice of acupuncture is based on both observation and scientific research that have been in continuous evolution for thousands of years. Unlike modern scientific medical practice, which has only been present for a few hundred years, this extremely long history of acupuncture has provided a milieu of interpretations that contributes to disagreements in how to perceive the effectiveness of this technique. Although the science of acupuncture was originally based on meticulous categorization from observable evidence, a large metaphysical tradition formed around the practice and became a popular mechanism to explain the beneficial effects of this treatment. There remains, however, a paired scientific understanding and inquiry around the precise neurobiological mechanism of acupuncture: in the West as well as in China and globally.[6] For the purposes of this discussion, the scientific neurophysiologic understanding of acupuncture as a treatment modality is presented in this article. There are vast data for this discussion, and a scientific imperative to study and understand modalities through measurable parameters.

ACUPUNCTURE IS APPLIED ANATOMY

Acupuncture points have distinct anatomic underpinnings that can be understood based on the integral homeostasis of living organisms. These points were found by trial and error as well as by being in the vicinity of important neurovascular structures (bleeding from these areas was crucial traditionally).[7] Acupuncture points have since been linked to "lines" or "meridians" that partially relate to anatomic similarities, such as major nerve pathways, dermatomes, sclerotomes, or sensations related to axon anatomy. These lines or meridians are described by metaphysical explanations as well as the grouping of points that was observed to have similar effects on various body systems.[8] From the point of view of traditional Western-based medicine, the acupuncture points do not follow precise anatomic counterparts. However, using common names for these points allows for a universal understanding. Thus, in the scientific and medical approach to acupuncture, the same names have been preserved, despite the added complexity that these points are assembled in ways that are not always clearly logical from the anatomic framework (**Fig. 1**).

Acupuncture can be described as a tool that helps modify the endogenous homeostasis of the various body systems of an organism. The major anatomic structures modified by acupuncture include nerves (sensory, motor, and autonomic), blood vessels, fascial sheets, and lymphatic beds. Acupuncture exerts its effects by modifying the function of these anatomic structures and thus changing body homeostasis.[7] For the purposes of this article, each of the following anatomic areas will be individually

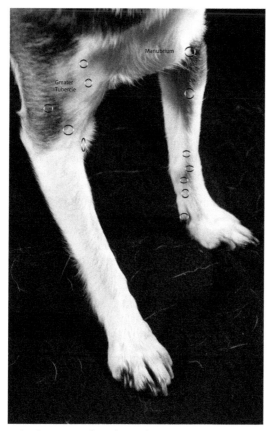

Fig. 1. Neuro-anatomic placement of LU channel acupuncture points of the forelimb. (*Courtesy of* Bonnie Wright, DVM, DACVAA. Johnstown, CO.)

described in order to emphasize the anatomic and physiologic rationale behind acupuncture treatment:

- Cutaneous structures: nerves, fascia, and microcirculation
- Corridor structures: axons, fascia, lymphatic channels and nodes, and myotendinous structures
- Spinal structures: somatic, autonomic, and spinal arc reflexes
- Central structures: brain, brainstem

CUTANEOUS STRUCTURES

Histologic analysis has demonstrated that acupuncture points contain somatic anatomic structures, such as free nerve endings, encapsulated cutaneous receptors, and musculotendinous sensory receptors (muscle spindles and Golgi tendon organs). Despite an ongoing search for a basis to the concept of "Chi, or energy," no other structure aside from fascia has been consistently identified in these tissues.[7]

Acupuncture points are found in cutaneous regions that are highly innervated.[6] They are found where groups of nerves emerge through foramens, muscle, and fascia, where they branch or join, and where they attenuate distally.[9] These nerve fibers are made up of Aα, Aβ Aδ (myelinated), and C (nonmyelinated) fibers as well as autonomic fibers.[7]

In general, a prevalence of myelinated somatic sensory fibers is seen near acupuncture points, with most being Aβ and Aδ, with the exception of motor or Golgi-tendon points. Although there is often a focus in acupuncture research on understanding the modification of high-threshold (pain sensing) nerve types, there are also studies surrounding the low-threshold mechanoreceptors (LTMRs).[10] Acupuncture needle placement is rarely painful, and it is likely that many of the sensations associated with it (such as warmth, cool, pressure, and movement) are actually secondary to LTMR activation more than nociceptor activation.

These peripheral anatomic structures help to explain why neuromodulation is the primary mechanism of action for acupuncture, and this is true for the skin as well as for peripheral nerve bundles. Acupuncture stimulates afferent nerve fibers. Afferent stimulation is present for both manual acupuncture as well as electroacupuncture. Both manual stimulation and electrical stimulation stimulate all 4 types of nerve fibers: Aα, Aβ, Aδ, and C fibers, although these occur with different discharge frequencies.[11] Interaction with these various nerve fibers creates a variety of sensory sensations in response to the needle penetration. Terms such as heaviness and distention are associated with myelinated Aβ and Aδ fibers as well as sensory units, such as Golgi tendon organs and muscle spindles. Soreness, sharpness, aching, coolness, and warmth are associated with pain fibers, such as C fibers and Aδ fibers found in regions rich in these cutaneous nociceptors.[12] Acupuncture also benefits from the reflex activity of the axons, providing a cutaneous autocrine response at the afferent sensory nerves, simultaneous with the signal traveling along the prodromal nerve pathway, and potentially providing an anatomic key to the sensation of energy moving along meridians.[7]

When evaluating the similarities and divergent characteristics between the recognized acupuncture points on the body, an important consideration is the global position of the point on the organism. For example, distal points tend to have greater homeostatic effects, such as regulation of immune function, organ function, and sympathetic/parasympathetic balance. This observation is partially explained because autonomic fiber density is increased in the distal limbs. Many of these peripheral autonomic fibers are sympathetic, monoaminergic fibers, which are a staple of neurologic and immune homeostasis.[7]

Proximal points tend to have a greater musculoskeletal influence, except for points adjunct to the spinal cord, which provide neuromodulation in additional to musculoskeletal modification. More proximal points are found where deep nerve and fascia penetrate muscle bellies, such as between the longissimus and iliocostalis paraspinal groups.

Another important consideration for the divergent nature of proximal axillary and distal appendicular points is the skin type represented in these regions. There are distinct physiologic differences between haired skin (over most of the body) and nonhaired (glabrous) skin, found particularly on the feet of quadrupeds. Nonhaired skin encodes complex information about touch, including discrimination of location, shape, and type of stimulus. A greater arousal and sympathetic modulations are possible from these regions, whereas axillary points may favor parasympathetic flow.

Receptors in nonhaired skin include Merkel cells (static touch), Ruffini corpuscles (stretch), Meissner corpuscles (movement), and Pacinian corpuscles (vibration). Haired skin has a decreased discrimination role compared with nonhaired skin. However, it has an important affective role directly contributing to emotive, calming, and soothing brain centers. In haired skin, there are specialized Merkel cells conveying information on tissue deformation, movement of tissue on a deeper level owing to nerve fibers wrapping around hair follicles, and specialized unmyelinated, slowly conducted LTMRs that convey touch sensation.[9] Understanding the neural encoding of cutaneous receptors provides compelling insight into the observed unique characteristics of individual acupuncture points, because a vast array of sensory information is coded by the activation of a combination low-threshold receptors and nociceptors by an acupuncture needle.

Acupuncture points are described according to the underpinning physiology and the interaction between the somatic and autonomic components of the "neural acupuncture unit" (NAU). Modulating local and ascending (afferent) signals are responsible for the neurologic complexity seen with punctate stimulation of these regions.[6] The description of the NAU needs to include the nerves, their cutaneous receptors, but also the neurochemical milieu and microcirculatory transportation sharing this space.

Nerve endings exist in a context of cellular and vascular structures, including mast cells, endothelial cells, keratinocytes, fascia, sympathetically rich microcirculation, and lymphatic vessels. This cellular complex releases many neurotransmitters that can be excitatory or inhibitory.[12] Homeostasis involves the summation of these inputs, and acupuncture relies as much on this chemical milieu as it does the direct interaction with nerves.[7]

At the most basic, the NAU can be described as a triad, with nerve-ending, associated mast cells and capillaries.[9] There are receptors associated with both the nerve ending and the mast cells that convey the properties of detecting different types of stimulus, such as mechanical, thermal, electrical, and chemical. Transient receptor potential (TRP) channels are well recognized to serve in these roles and are directly modified by acupuncture treatment.[13] The mast cells, which serve as front-line immune sentries, also show activation through TRP channels, purines, and immunoglobulins. At the point of an acupuncture needle, purines and histamines are major contributors to the local response as well as the spreading of this focal signal into a systemic and homeostasis-modifying effect.

Fibroblasts are also present in the NAU, which speaks to the ubiquitous presence of fascia in the body. It is found in all body tissues and is present as the intima in organs.[14] Once considered inert, because of scientific studies on the mechanisms of acupuncture, the fascia has been credited with an important role in fluid movement through tissues, immune modulation, musculoskeletal programming, proprioception, and cancer.[12] Paired with this discovery is the histologic evidence that acupuncture works directly through stimulation of cutaneous fascia, making this the mechanical link between the acupuncture needle and the nervous system.[15]

With insertion and rotation of an acupuncture needle, collagen fibrils pull on the associated fibroblast, causing remodeling of the cellular structure within 10 minutes, as well as release of purines from both the fibroblasts and the mast cells that are caught up in this wave of mechanical stretching. The mechanical stretching of fibroblasts is followed within 90 minutes by increased mechanotransduction and upregulation of genes related to muscle and sensory homeostasis. Unlike other forms of collagen deformation, such as massage and stretching, the acupuncture needle creates a microscopic "whorl" of collage within the connective tissue, which may result in a biochemical modification and changes in connective tissue tension regulation that can last for hours to days, as compared with other forms of intervention.[14]

Other cutaneous structures in the vicinity of the peripheral nerve terminal, such as mast cells, endothelial cells, and migrating inflammatory cells, play a significant role in the peripheral effects of acupuncture.[12,16]

CORRIDOR STRUCTURES

Fascia, lymphatics, and the axon reflex are considered "corridor structures" for their roles more distant from the initial peripheral activity that occurs in proximity to an acupuncture point receiving input. The "corridor" functions to connect the peripheral point of action to the rest of the body.

Changes in the "loose" connective tissue of the body have a dramatic influence on fluid movement through the tissues, because the appendicular connective tissue is the home of the lymphatic system. The lymphatic system plays a critical role in immune homeostasis, as is demonstrated by the coalescing of lymphocytes and other immune cells into the lymph nodes along these lymphatic chains. Thus, the fibroblasts, and by extension, acupuncture are integral into immune homeostasis as well as neurologic processing homeostasis.[15,17]

When an acupuncture needle is placed, a dynamic and self-sustaining change occurs in the fascia, and this can be identified microscopically, but also by measuring chemical mediators and genetic transcription. This local change in the fascia likely ripples along the fascial network of an organism, creating far-reaching change. Of note, this impact also self-sustains, because fibroblasts will pull on their neighbors, changing the neurochemistry of adjacent structures and creating a chain reaction that spreads the signal over both space and time.[14]

The fascia is also integral to the movement of fluid through the tissues. Furthermore, organs rich in fascia as well as appendicular structures are really serving as fluid highways and even have regulatory capacities over the movement of these fluids.[15] Fascial structures have also been found to have significant independent innervation, allowing them to provide a proprioceptive, body-wide sense of awareness. Also, they are an active component in the coordination of movement, protecting joints from uncoordinated stresses as well as integrating the communication along similar muscle groups (such as coordinating extension between the quadriceps and gastrocnemius muscle).[12]

Thus, fascia provides a critical component of the efficacy of acupuncture treatment. In the periphery, this is primarily tied into the microcirculation and microscopic nerve and vasodilatory influences. Along the body, this is tied into a macroscopic structure bringing together nerve and motor communication, and body awareness and providing for the delivery and removal of life-sustaining fluids to the extravascular body compartments.

The afferent axons of the neurons also run through the corridor compartment and play a large role in acupuncture treatment as well as laser treatment along acupuncture points.[18] An antidromal axon reflex is present in sensory fibers. The primary recipients of this high-speed nerve input are mast cells, sweat glands, and blood vessels, which are all involved in the contribution and response to acupuncture treatment. The axon reflex activates autocrine groups along the stimulated axon, causing some of the sensation associated with the stimulation of acupuncture points. The axon reflex may be the mechanism that identifies acupuncture channels.[6]

Included with corridor structures are other sensory components: muscle spindles and Golgi-tendon organs. NAUs have been subdivided, based on the relative predominance of receptor types, into 3 types: muscle-spindle-rich NAUs, cutaneous-receptor-rich NAUs, and tendon-organ-rich NAUs.[8] The cutaneous NAU was covered in the previous section; in this section, the spindle-rich and tendon-rich NAUs are discussed, because these tend to be located more proximally, along the "corridor" between the cutaneous and deep structures.

A structure that is often described in the spinal or central compartment but is actually a component of the peripheral nervous system is the cell body of the dorsal root ganglion. Managing the receptor populations, microtubular arrays, and ion channel representation, the nerve cell body is integrally involved in the signals ascending from the peripheral tissues to the spinal cord. An important contributor to the analgesia effects of acupuncture are purines, released in peripheral tissues during acupuncture needle stimulation. These neurotransmitters create transcriptional changes at the nerve cell body in the dorsal root ganglion, resulting in modification of the pain signals at the level of the axon distal to the dorsal root ganglion.[19,20]

Departing from the neurologic and fascial components of the corridor structures affected by acupuncture, direct effects on motor units are also a component of acupuncture treatment. This commonly targeted benefit of acupuncture is also shared by techniques known as "dry needling" done by physical therapists and acupuncturists alike. Several named acupuncture points exist over motor units that can contain sensory motor fibers. The sensation of needling these regions is characterized by cramping-type pain, and much of this signal is carried via $A\gamma$ and $A\delta$ nerve fibers.[6] Trigger points can also occur in motor regions not directly related to acupuncture points. However, 1 category of acupuncture points is known as Ah Shi points, or painful points. Ah Shi Points will most often be trigger point regions, because trigger points are algogenic regions and contribute to generalized pain sensitization.[21]

For pain conditions, trigger points in muscles are a common and important component of treatment, in addition to named points that are treated in proximity to the painful site, proximal and distal to the pain along the nervous system, and points that are primarily homeostatic as well as paired points on the opposite limbs. Whether these are seen as Ah Shi points or simply "dry needling" is clinically unimportant. Whatever the viewpoint, the approach is to disinhibit muscles that are restricted by poor blood flow, algogenic substances, and reduced function. Disinhibition is accomplished through inserting needles into the damaged, contracted region to bring in nutritive blood flow, reduce pain, restore function, and collaborate with neighboring muscle groupings.[18]

In addition to release of trigger points from muscle groups, acupuncture can modify the sensory and reflex-loop portion of the motor unit. The sensory portion of muscles is the muscle spindles, and these are located diffusely throughout motor units. These sensory structures are more replete in muscles that have a larger proprioceptive role. Acupuncture over muscles can interact with the muscle spindle units, modifying the sensations experienced by the muscles, but also interacting with the reflex arcs that increase or decrease muscle contraction in the presence of stretch or fibrosis.

Golgi tendon organs are deep structures, and like the muscle spindle points, they have a role in managing musculoskeletal conditions whereby pain, damage, or musculotendinous shortening have taken place. Needle placement in NAUs with strong tendon input will feed into the reflex relaxation of the associated myotendinous structures and cause an immediate reduction to local pain. There will also be a long-term reduction in wind up, and amplification of soft tissue immobility.[7]

Before leaving the corridor structures, a caveat of acupuncture needling should be mentioned. Any 1 acupuncture point may generate input from both cutaneous sources and deeper sources, such as trigger points, muscle spindles, and Golgi tendon organs. In general, data exist that deeper needling generates a greater biological response, so a summation of input from a combination of both cutaneous and deeper structures is recommended. At the same time, any needled point carries the cutaneous sensory and fascial input. This input is part of the reason acupuncture performs poorly in placebo-controlled studies, because some biological response will be seen whether a true acupuncture point is used, versus any other point on the body. The responses to sham versus verum acupuncture have been shown to differ in magnitude, because acupuncture points are universally located in regions with potent neurochemical underpinnings, but differences in magnitude are difficult to detect in clinical studies.[22]

SPINAL STRUCTURES

The dorsal horn of the spinal cord is the receiving zone for afferent impulses ascending from the periphery. Significant diversity of receptors, pain fibers, and neurochemical compounds contributes to the magnitude and type of signal seen at the level of the dorsal horn. At this level, the signal is transduced to spinothalamic tracts that ascend to the thalamus. At this level, there is a vast opportunity to modify this signal with acupuncture.

At the level of the dorsal horn, a variety of mechanisms can modify the likelihood that the signal will cross the synapse and create an action potential propagating the painful stimulus to the second order neurons. Signal modulation occurs through changes in GABA, serotonin, norepinephrine, calcitonin gene-related peptide, substance P, endorphins, and cannabinoids. Acupuncture effects emanating from the periphery have been shown to exert at least some modification on each of these neurotransmitters in various laboratory studies.[6,23–25]

In addition to the modifications possible at the first synapse, the topography of the spinal cord provides for interneurons that can inhibit or amplify the incoming afferent signal. Concepts such as diffuse noxious inhibitory control are being used to assess amplified pain states as well as detect therapies, such as acupuncture, that work to decrease central pain amplification.[26] Inhibitory Control of pain can be modified by the local neurochemical milieu, but also by descending input from the midbrain. Acupuncture input has also been shown to aid in the modification of descending inhibitory mechanisms, and this method of testing the nervous system may significantly improve the clinical data needed to demonstrate acupuncture efficacy.[27]

In the dorsal horn of the spinal cord and present in all structures within the blood-brain barrier are glia. Glia surround each synapse and participate in specific synaptic activities. The glia act as structural and inflammatory cells of the nervous system. They are involved in sleep, mood, pain amplification, pain suppression, tolerance, and addiction. Acupuncture has been shown to influence the activity of glia, potentially reversing some of the negative effects of glial stimulators (like the opioids) and decreasing the long-term central neuroinflammation resulting from pain and opioid treatments alike.[28]

The somatotropic layout of the spinal cord is integral to the function of acupuncture to modify deep tissues and organs. Deeper tissues can be modified by interacting with somatic sites that share the same spinal innervation network. Examples of this used by modern medicine include "sea bands" for nausea (over PC-6 acupuncture point) and electrical stimulation over the tibial nerve (KI-3 acupuncture point) to aid in urinary retention.[29]

Modification of autonomic outflow is most likely near accessible portions of the sympathetic chain and parasympathetic ganglia. Examples of sympathetic proximity include the cervicothoracic junction (start of the sympathetic chain) and the lumbosacral junction (sacral sympathetic outflow). Examples of parasympathetic ganglia are in the thoracolumbar region (stellate) and at the thoracic inlet (cranial cervical ganglion). In addition to modification of autonomic function through the vagal nerve, acupuncture can influence sympathetic outflow and certain points, and parasympathetic outflow at others.[30] Spinal reflex arcs in addition to the modification of sympathetic/parasympathetic balance more globally have been shown to contribute to some of the organ effects seen with acupuncture, such as regulation of cardiac activity.[31]

BRAIN STRUCTURES

Studying acupuncture's central effects has traditionally been limited to laboratory animals, because of the invasiveness of such studies. Decades of data show influences on neurotransmitters, especially endogenous opioids. The reliance of laboratory models of pain has not answered the lingering questions about why acupuncture appears so effective for mood and behavior. However, neuroimaging studies have provided vast amounts of data, although there remains controversy as to how to value and interpret these data. In general, imaging studies have shown complex activation and deactivation of many areas of the brain. In general, verum acupuncture needles have shown a larger effect than sham, and having a deep needling treatment, with adequate tissue grab (deqi) appears important. The periaqueductal gray and ventrolateral medulla show consistent responses to acupuncture for pain.[32]

SUMMARY

The author's hope is that she has convincingly laid out the myriad of ways that acupuncture has been clearly demonstrated to help modify pain sensing. In doing so, the author hopes she has also dispelled some of the myths that have kept the medical community from acknowledging acupuncture's efficacy in treating pain. The Veterinary community is at the threshold of more universal utilization of physical medicine modalities, buoyed by reams of physiologic and clinical data. The silver lining to the opioid crisis is that it his hastened this change. Although learning this new skill will take practitioners some time and effort, the benefits of doing so clearly outweigh the costs. To finish, the author provides a quote from the white paper: *Acupuncture's Role is Solving the Opioid Epidemic from November 2017*:

The United States (U.S.) is facing a national opioid epidemic, and medical systems are in need of non-pharmacologic strategies that can be employed to decrease the public's opioid dependence. Acupuncture has emerged as a powerful, evidence-based, safe, cost-effective, and available treatment modality suitable to meeting this need. Acupuncture has been shown to be effective for the management of numerous types of pain conditions, and mechanisms of action for acupuncture have been described and are understandable from biomedical, physiologic perspectives. Further, acupuncture's cost-effectiveness can dramatically decrease health care expenditures, both from the standpoint of treating acute pain and through avoiding addiction to opioids that requires costly care, destroys quality of life, and can lead to fatal overdose. Numerous federal regulatory agencies have advised or mandated that healthcare systems and providers offer non-pharmacologic treatment options for pain. Acupuncture stands out as the most evidence-based, immediately available choice to fulfil these calls. Acupuncture can safely, easily, and cost-effectively be incorporated into hospital settings as diverse as the emergency department, labor and delivery suites, and neonatal intensive care units to treat a variety of commonly seen pain conditions. Acupuncture is already being successfully and meaningfully utilized by the Veterans Administration and various branches of the U.S. Military, in some studies demonstrably decreasing the volume of opioids prescribed when included in care.[33]

REFERENCES

1. Roeckel L-A, Le Coz G-M, Gaveriaux-Ruff C, et al. Opioid-induced hyperalgesia: cellular and molecular mechanisms. Neuroscience 2016;338:160–82.
2. Plein LM, Rittner HL. Opioids and the immune system–friend or foe. Br J Pharmacol 2018;175(14):2717–25.
3. KuKanich B. Outpatient oral analgesics in dogs and cats beyond nonsteroidal antiinflammatory drugs: an evidence-based approach. Vet Clin North Am Small Anim Pract 2013;43(5):1109–25.
4. HeatherTick AN. Evidence-based nonpharmacologic strategies for comprehensive pain care: the consortium pain task force white paper. Explore (NY) 2018; 14:177–211.
5. Chen WG, Niemtzow RC, Belfer I, et al. Acupuncture versus opioids for pain relief: an expert discussion. Med Acupunct 2018;30(6):290–5.
6. Cheng KJ. Neurobiological mechanisms of acupuncture for some common illnesses: a clinician's perspective. J Acupunct Meridian Stud 2014;7:105–14.
7. Zhao Z-Q. Neural mechanism underlying acupuncture analgesia. Prog Neurobiol 2008;85(4):355–75.
8. Zhang ZJ, Wang XM, McAlonan GM. Neural acupuncture unit: a new concept for interpreting effects and mechanisms of acupuncture. Evid Based Complement Alternat Med 2012;2012.
9. Tao ZL. The progress of the morphological research on the acupoint. Zhen Ci Yan Jiu 1989;14(4):397–402 [in Chinese].
10. Zimmerman A, Bai L, Ginty DD. (14AD). The gentle touch of mammalian skin. Science 346(6212):950–4.
11. Kagitani F, Uchida S, Hotta H. Afferent nerve fibers and acupuncture. Auton Neurosci 2010;157(1–2):2–8.
12. Wall PD, McMahon SB, Koltzenburg M. Wall and Melzack's textbook of pain. 6th edition. Saunders; 2013.
13. Huang M, Wang X, Xing B, et al. Critical roles of TRPV2 channels, histamine H1 and adenosine A1 receptors in the initiation of acupoint signals for acupuncture analgesia. Sci Rep 2018;8(1):1–11.
14. Adstrum S, Hedley G, Schleip R, et al. Defining the fascial system. J Bodyw Mov Ther 2017;21(1):173–7.
15. Gray W. Anisotropic tissue motion induced by acupuncture needling along intermuscular connective tissue. Planes 2014;20(4):290–4.
16. Yin N, Yang H, Yao W, et al. Mast cells and nerve signal conduction in acupuncture. Evid Based Complement Alternat Med 2018;2018. https://doi.org/10.1155/2018/3524279.
17. Langevin HM, Nedergaard M, Howe A. Cellular control of the connective tissue matrix tension. J Cell Biochem 2013;114(8):1–11. https://doi.org/10.1002/jcb.24521.CELLULAR.
18. Wang L, Hu L, Grygorczyk R, et al. Modulation of extracellular ATP content of mast cells and DRG neurons by irradiation: studies on underlying mechanism of low-level-laser therapy. Mediators Inflamm 2015;2015:630361.

19. Tang Y, Yin H, Liu J, et al. P2X receptors and acupuncture analgesia. Brain Res Bull 2018. https://doi.org/10.1016/j.brainresbull.2018.10.015.
20. Weng ZJ, Wu LY, Zhou CL, et al. Effect of electroacupuncture on P2X3receptor regulation in the peripheral and central nervous systems of rats with visceral pain caused by irritable bowel syndrome. Purinergic Signal 2015;11(3):321–9.
21. Dommerholt J. Dry needling—peripheral and central considerations. J Man Manip Ther 2011;19(4):223–7.
22. Scheffold BE, Hsieh CL, Litscher G. Neuroimaging and neuromonitoring effects of electro and manual acupuncture on the central nervous system: a literature review and analysis. Evid Based Complement Alternat Med 2015;2015. https://doi.org/10.1155/2015/641742.
23. Jiang SW, Lin YW, Hsieh CL. Electroacupuncture at Hua Tuo Jia Ji acupoints reduced neuropathic pain and increased GABAAreceptors in rat spinal cord. Evid Based Complement Alternat Med 2018;2018. https://doi.org/10.1155/2018/8041820.
24. Villarreal Santiago M, Tumilty S, Mącznik A, et al. Does acupuncture alter pain-related functional connectivity of the central nervous system? A systematic review. J Acupunct Meridian Stud 2016;9(4):167–77.
25. Yuan X-C, Wang Q, Su W, et al. Electroacupuncture potentiates peripheral CB2 receptor-inhibited chronic pain in a mouse model of knee osteoarthritis. J Pain Res 2018;11:2797–808.
26. Cathcart S, Winefield AH, Rolan Phd P, et al. Reliability of temporal summation and diffuse noxious inhibitory control. Pain Res Manag 2009;14:433–8. Available at: https://www.ncbi.nlm.nih.gov/pmc/articles/PMC2807770/pdf/prm14433.pdf.
27. Kong JT, Schnyer RN, Johnson KA, et al. Understanding central mechanisms of acupuncture analgesia using dynamic quantitative sensory testing: a review. Evid Based Complement Alternat Med 2013;2013. https://doi.org/10.1155/2013/187182.
28. Lin L, Skakavac N, Lin X, et al. Acupuncture-induced analgesia: the role of microglial inhibition. Cell Transplant 2016;25(4):621–8. https://doi.org/10.3727/096368916X690872.
29. Macpherson H, Coeytaux RR, Davis RT, et al. Unanticipated insights into biomedicine from the study of acupuncture. J Altern Complement Med 2016;22(2):101–7.
30. Lim HD, Kim MH, Lee CY, et al. Anti-inflammatory effects of acupuncture stimulation via the vagus nerve. PLoS One 2016;11(3):1–15.
31. Li P, Tjen-A-Looi SC, Guo Z-L, et al. Long-loop pathways in cardiovascular electroacupuncture responses. J Appl Physiol 1985 2009;106(2):620–30.
32. Knudsen L, Petersen GL, Norskov KN, et al. Review of neuroimaging studies related to pain modulation. Scand J Pain 2018;2(3):108–20.
33. Fan AY, Miller DW, Bolash B, et al. Acupuncture's role in solving the opioid epidemic: evidence, cost-effectiveness, and care availability for acupuncture as a primary, non-pharmacologic method for pain relief and management-white paper 2017. J Integr Med 2017;15(6):411–25.

Locoregional Anesthesia of the Head

Ana C. Castejón-González, DVM, PhD*, Alexander M. Reiter, Dipl. Tzt., Dr med vet

KEYWORDS

- Nerve block • Splash block • Infiltration • Local anesthetic • Dental surgery
- Oral surgery • Ocular surgery • Auricular surgery

KEY POINTS

- Locoregional anesthesia provides perioperative analgesia, reduces the intraoperative anesthetic requirements, and decreases the postoperative need for systemic analgesics.
- Locoregional anesthesia techniques are relatively easy to accomplish, but cadaver practice is recommended to enable the veterinarian to feel comfortable and master the techniques.
- Locoregional anesthesia can be considered for many surgical procedures of the head; however, understanding the patient's anatomy and the techniques' limitations is important to avoid complications and obtain the best possible outcome.

INTRODUCTION

The recent concern among veterinarians associated with the "opioid crisis" and the shortage in the availability of opioids in the veterinary market demands more than ever the use of multimodal strategies for pain management.[1] The International Veterinary Academy of Pain Management and the American College of Veterinary Anesthesia and Analgesia advocate for the use of locoregional anesthesia with nonopioids or opioid-sparing anesthetic protocols. Locoregional anesthesia provides perioperative analgesia, reduces the intraoperative anesthetic requirements, and decreases the postoperative need for systemic analgesics.[2–9]

The innervation of the globe and periocular tissues, nasal and oral cavity, and ear and face is complex with areas innervated by multiple nerves or nerves that cannot be safely blocked. However, locoregional anesthesia can be performed for several procedures such as tooth extractions or root canal therapy without the need for intraoperative systemic analgesics. The use of opioids can be reduced or avoided if appropriate locoregional techniques are used for certain procedures of the oral cavity, nasal cavity, eye, or ear. Protocols with α2-agonists, lidocaine, ketamine, and nerve blocks

---

Department of Clinical Sciences and Advanced Medicine, School of Veterinary Medicine, University of Pennsylvania, 3900 Delancey Street, Philadelphia, PA 19104, USA
* Corresponding author.
E-mail address: anacaste@upenn.edu

Vet Clin Small Anim 49 (2019) 1041–1061
https://doi.org/10.1016/j.cvsm.2019.07.011
0195-5616/19/© 2017 Elsevier Inc. All rights reserved.

are alternatives to analgesic protocols with opioids.[1] Contraindications for locoregional anesthesia are the presence of neoplasia, infection, or severe inflammation in the area of injection.[3,9]

EQUIPMENT

The equipment necessary for administration of locoregional anesthesia is minimal: hypodermic needles, 1- to 3-mL syringes, and local anesthetic solutions. For intraoral nerve blocks (through the mucosa) the authors use 27-gauge long (1$\frac{1}{4}$ inch) or short (½ inch) needles, and for extraoral nerve blocks (through skin) 22- to 25-gauge needles (⅝ inch to 1 inch long). The use of needles with smaller bore reduces potential damage to neurovascular structures.[9] Some authors recommend the use of a 20-gauge intravenous catheter instead of a needle to perform the maxillary nerve block through the infraorbital canal.[4] A 22-gauge spinal needle is frequently used for analgesia of the retrobulbar space.[10–12] In small dogs and cats, hypodermic needles are long enough to reach the targeted area.[12]

REGIONAL ANESTHESIA (NERVE BLOCKS)

The selection of the local anesthetic to be used is based on the type and length of the procedure. For shorter procedures or procedures that start shortly after the injection, short-acting drugs with a rapid onset of effect might be a better choice (**Table 1**). The authors prefer bupivacaine for nerve blocks because of its long duration of action that provides pain control during the procedure and during the immediate postoperative period. If the effect weans off, the nerve block can be repeated intraoperatively or just before recovery from anesthesia. A mixture of 2% lidocaine and 0.5% bupivacaine has been used in an attempt to have the benefits of both drugs (quick onset of the lidocaine and extended duration of the bupivacaine), but the benefit of this combination is not clear.[12,13] The optimal volume to be used for each nerve block has not been established; therefore, the selection of the volume is based on previously published reports and the experience of the clinician (**Table 2**). The veterinarian should calculate the total maximum dose that can be safely administered at a given time (**Box 1**). This is extremely important if multiple nerve blocks are performed at the same time and

Table 1				
Local anesthetics commonly used in locoregional anesthesia				
Local Anesthetic	Maximum Total Dose (mg/kg)	Onset	Duration	Comments
Bupivacaine	D: 2 C: 1–2	Slow 5–10 min	Long 180–480 min	Possibly longer duration of the analgesic effect (24–72 h)[40] Severe cardiac depression reported in a cat after administration of a nerve block at 1.16 mg/kg[38]
Lidocaine	D: 5 C: 3	Fast 2–5 min	Short 60–120 min	
Mepivacaine	D: 5 C: 1.5	Fast 2–5 min	Short 90–180 min	
Ropivacaine	D: 3	Fast 5–10 min	Long 180–480 min	

Abbreviations: C, cat; D, dog.

Table 2
Suggested volumes of local anesthetics for nerve blocks of the oral cavity

Oral cavity[a]	Volume (mL)
Cats and small dogs	0.1–0.3
Medium-sized dogs	0.3–0.5
Large dogs	0.5–0.8
Giant dogs	0.8–1.0
Eye	
Retrobulbar nerve block	1–2
Peribulbar nerve block	2–4
Ear	
Auriculotemporal nerve block	0.5–1.5[31]
Great auricular nerve block	0.5–1.5[31]

[a] The volume injected into the infraorbital canal or the mandibular canal is usually smaller than the volume used for the maxillary or inferior alveolar nerve block. The volume for the major palatine nerve block should not exceed 0.1 mL in cats and small dogs and 0.2 to 0.4 mL in larger dogs.

the patient is small.[6,9,14] For instance, the maximum volume of 0.5% bupivacaine that can be administered at the same time in a 5-kg dog will be 2 mL (maximum dose 2 mg/kg of bupivacaine, concentration 5 mg/mL). Therefore, if the objective is to block the 4 quadrants of the oral cavity, each block should not exceed 0.5 mL. Since the dog in this example is small, there is no need to administer 0.5 mL for each block, and it would likely be sufficient to use only 0.3 mL per nerve block.

NERVE BLOCKS OF THE ORAL AND NASAL CAVITIES

There are 5 nerve blocks that can be used in the oral cavity: maxillary, infraorbital, major palatine, inferior alveolar, and middle mental.[3,9,14–16] We recommend bilateral

Box 1
Check list

- Calculate the maximum volume that can be given in a patient based on weight. If more volume is needed to assure diffusion of the solution in a larger area, the volume can be increased by adding saline solution.
- Calculate the volume needed to block the nerve.
- Select the smallest needle that allows for reaching the target area and causing minimal trauma.
- Select the local anesthetic drug and verify its concentration on the bottle label.
- Avoid areas of neoplasia, infection, or inflammation in the area of injection.
- Identify the anatomic landmarks.
- Confirm extravascular injection of the solution by aspirating before injection of the local anesthetic.
- If blood is aspirated, retrieve the needle from the tissue and apply digital pressure. Use a new syringe and needle to make another attempt. If blood is aspirated again, do not use that nerve block or make another attempt later.

nerve blocks if the area to be operated on is in the midline of the oral cavity (incisive area, palate, and symphysis).

Neuroanatomy

The sensory innervation of the oral cavity is provided by the maxillary and mandibular branches of the trigeminal nerve. The maxillary nerve runs ventral to the eye. In the pterygopalatine fossa, it sends out off the pterygopalatine nerve, and its branches provide sensation to the nasal cavity (caudal nasal nerve) and hard and soft palate (major and minor palatine nerves). The maxillary nerve enters the infraorbital canal at the maxillary foramen to become the infraorbital nerve, which already sends out the caudal superior alveolar branches in the pterygopalatine fossa, the middle superior alveolar branches within the infraorbital canal, and the rostral superior alveolar branches before exiting its canal at the infraorbital foramen. The rostral superior alveolar branches continue into the incisivomaxillary canal that runs in the maxilla. In cats, the middle superior alveolar branches also arise from the infraorbital nerve in the pterygopalatine fossa. The caudal, middle, and rostral superior alveolar branches supply the teeth. The infraorbital nerve continues rostrally to supply the rostral lip and nose with its labial and nasal branches.[3,17]

The mandibular nerve has sensory and motor innervation. The branches with interest for locoregional anesthesia are the auriculotemporal nerve that supply the ear, the parotid salivary gland, skin on the side of the face, and the inferior alveolar nerve. The inferior alveolar nerve runs on the medial aspect of the pterygoid muscle and enters the mandibular canal at the mandibular foramen. Within the canal, it sends out the caudal, middle, and rostral alveolar branches that supply the teeth. The inferior alveolar nerve exits the mandibular canal through the caudal, middle, and rostral mental foramina, sending out the branches with the same name that supply the rostral lip and oral mucosa.[3,17] Because of the complex and collateral innervation of the skin, buccal mucosa, and intermandibular space, it is impossible to desensitize completely the oral and nasal cavities (**Table 3**).[3,4,17–19]

Maxillary Nerve Block

The maxillary nerve block desensitizes the maxilla, incisive bone, palate, maxillary teeth, gingiva, oral mucosa, nasal mucosa (partially), and skin on the same side.[2–4,9,14,16,18] The objective is to place the local anesthetic solution in the pterygopalatine fossa around the maxillary nerve before it enters the infraorbital canal.

- Intraoral approach caudal to the maxilla
  - The needle is bent about 8 to 10 mm away from its tip at an angle of approximately 45°. This is done with the help of the needle cap to maintain the sterility of the rest of the needle. This bend is a visual mark to avoid excessive insertion of the needle tip into the orbit (**Fig. 1**).
  - The needle is inserted through the mucosa caudal to the last molar tooth between its palatal and buccal aspects.
  - The needle is advanced dorsally into the pterygopalatine fossa for about 5 mm in a small dog or a cat and up to 1 cm in a large dog (**Fig. 2**).
- Intraoral approach through the infraorbital canal
  - The needle enters the infraorbital canal through the infraorbital foramen. The infraorbital foramen is located dorsal to the distal root of the maxillary third premolar tooth.
  - With the nondominant hand, the upper lip is retracted dorsally including the neurovascular bundle that exits from the infraorbital foramen.

Table 3
Recommended types of locoregional anesthesia for selected procedures of the head (oral cavity, eye, and ear)

Nerve Block	Nerves	Examples of Procedures
Maxillary nerve block	Maxillary nerve Infraorbital nerve Caudal, middle, and rostral superior alveolar dental nerves Pterygopalatine nerve Major and minor palatine nerves Caudal nasal nerve	Dental extractions (full maxillary quadrant) Soft- and hard-tissue biopsy Rhinoscopy, nasal biopsy Maxillectomy Palate surgery Lip and cheek resection Periodontal surgery Endodontic procedures Jaw fracture repair
Inferior alveolar nerve block	Inferior alveolar nerve Caudal, middle, and rostral inferior alveolar nerves Caudal, middle, and rostral mental nerves	Dental extraction (full mandibular quadrant) Mandibulectomy Periodontal surgery Endodontic procedure Jaw fracture repair
Caudal infraorbital nerve block	Infraorbital nerve; (possibly) caudal, middle, and rostral superior alveolar dental nerves	Dental extractions (premolar, canine, and incisor teeth) Soft- and hard-tissue biopsy of the oral cavity Maxillectomy (rostral or central) Periodontal surgery Endodontic procedures
Rostral infraorbital nerve block	Rostral portion of the infraorbital nerve, rostral alveolar superior dental nerve	Same procedures as for the maxillary nerve block but localized in the incisive area or up to the maxillary second premolar tooth
Mental nerve block	Middle mental nerve; possibly rostral portion of the inferior alveolar nerve, and rostral and middle alveolar inferior nerves	Laceration repair in the area of the mucosa in the rostral mandibular portion Gingivectomy Soft-tissue biopsy Not recommended for extraction or more invasive procedures
Major palatine nerve block	Major palatine nerve	Palatal surgery (do not use alone)
Retrobulbar block	Optic (II), oculomotor (III), trochlear (IV), ophthalmic (branch of V), abducens (VI), ciliary ganglion	Evisceration, enucleation, intraocular surgery
Peribulbar block	Terminal endings of the nerves around the ocular globe; if the local anesthetic solution diffuses to the retrobulbar area, it blocks the optic (II), oculomotor (III), trochlear (IV), ophthalmic (V3 branch of V), abducens (VI), and ciliary ganglion	Eyelid surgery, evisceration, enucleation, intraocular surgery

(continued on next page)

Table 3
(continued)

Nerve Block	Nerves	Examples of Procedures
Infiltration of eyelids	Terminal nerve endings at the injection site	Eyelid surgery; adjuvant with retrobulbar block for enucleation, evisceration
Great auricular nerve block[a]	Great auricular nerve (branch of the CN2)	Total ear canal ablation, surgery of the pinna
Auriculotemporal block[a]	Auriculotemporal nerve (branch of the mandibular nerve)	Total ear canal ablation, myringotomy, surgery of the pinna

[a] Use these two blocks together.
Data from Refs.[3,4,17,18]

- ○ The needle should penetrate the oral mucosa 5 mm (cat) to 10 mm (dog) rostral to the infraorbital foramen.
- ○ The needle is advanced into the infraorbital canal up to the pterygopalatine fossa (parallel to the hard palate to avoid injury of the eye). Instead of a needle, an intravenous catheter can be used to reach the pterygopalatine fossa, thus decreasing the risk of neurovascular damage (**Fig. 3**).[4,20]
- ○ The infraorbital canal in cats is very short (about 0.4 cm long).[3,21] The infraorbital foramen is located ventral to the orbit, medial to the rostral aspect of the zygomatic arch, and dorsal to the third premolar tooth. A double infraorbital foramen can be present, making the insertion of the needle into the canal more challenging.[22]

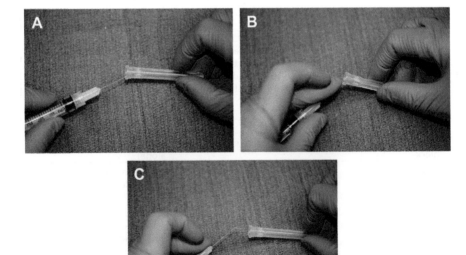

Fig. 1. Bending of a 27-gauge needle for maxillary nerve block. (*A*) The needle is introduced partially into the needle cap. (*B*) The middle finger holds the needle next to the point of bending and the needle cap is displaced toward the operator. (*C*) Bent needle at 45°. © 2019 Ana C. Castejón-González and Alexander M. Reiter.

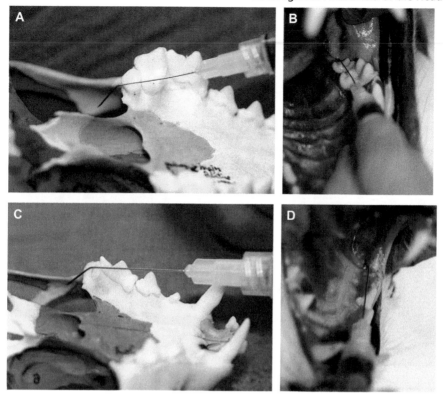

Fig. 2. Maxillary nerve block. (*A*) Position of the bent needle in a canine skull. (*B*) Placement of the needle in the pterygopalatine fossa in a dog. Avoid excessive insertion of the needle into the orbit. (*C*) Position of the bent needle in a feline skull. (*D*) Placement of the needle in the pterygopalatine fossa in a cat caudal to the first molar tooth. © 2019 Ana C. Castejón-González and Alexander M. Reiter.

- Extraoral approach caudal to the maxilla
  - The injection point for this approach is located in the skin caudal to the maxilla, ventral to the most rostral aspect of the zygomatic arch, and rostral to the coronoid process (**Fig. 4**).
  - The needle is advanced in a rostromedial direction into the pterygopalatine fossa.
  - If the needle touches the medial aspect of the orbit, it should be retracted a few millimeters.
- Transorbital approach
  - The needle is inserted in the conjunctiva of the lower eyelid, about 5 mm lateral to the medial canthus of the eye.
  - The needle is advanced until touching the bone of the caudal maxilla.[23]

A cadaveric study, comparing the extraoral approach caudal to the maxilla with the intraoral approach through the infraorbital canal, showed that the injection through the infraorbital canal has potentially more success in blocking the maxillary and the pterygopalatine nerves.[20]

Infraorbital Nerve Block

See also the previous section on maxillary nerve block through the infraorbital canal. The infraorbital nerve block desensitizes teeth, maxilla, incisive bone, upper lip, and

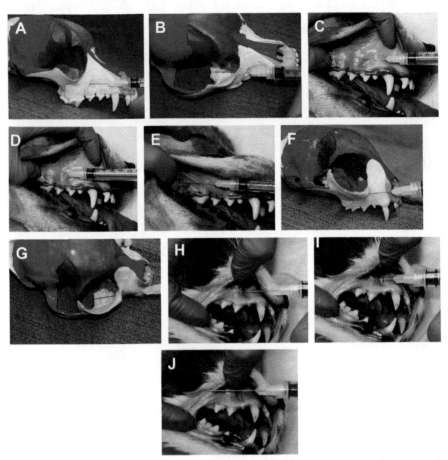

Fig. 3. Infraorbital nerve block. (*A*) Insertion of the needle parallel to the palate in a dog skull. The infraorbital foramen is dorsal to the distal root of the maxillary third premolar tooth. (*B*) The maxillary nerve can be reached if the needle is inserted deeply into the canal. The needle is advanced ventral to the eye. (*C*) The insertion of the needle in the oral mucosa is between the second and third premolar teeth. (*D*) Advancement of the needle into the canal. (*E*) The needle reaches the area of the molar teeth. Longer catheters can be used. (*F*) Insertion of the needle parallel to the palate in a cat skull. The infraorbital foramen is dorsal to the distal root of the maxillary third premolar tooth. (*G*) The maxillary nerve can be reached if the needle is inserted deeply into the canal. The needle is advanced ventral to the eye. (*H*) The insertion of the needle in the oral mucosa is between the second and third premolar teeth. (*I*) Advancement of the needle into the canal. (*J*) The needle reaches the area of the first molar tooth. Longer catheters can be used. © 2019 Ana C. Castejón-González and Alexander M. Reiter.

oral mucosa on the same side where the block is performed.[3,9,14] The extent of desensitization depends on how far caudal the local anesthetic has been administered. If the anesthetic is deposited in the pterygopalatine fossa, it will block all the superior alveolar branches that supply all teeth in that maxillary quadrant. If the drug is deposited in the middle or rostral part of the infraorbital canal, it will block the alveolar branches for the rostral premolar, canine, and incisor teeth.[13] Administration rostral to the infraorbital foramen will block only the branches that supply the rostral portion of the upper

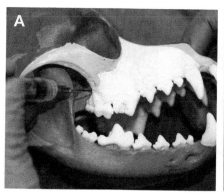
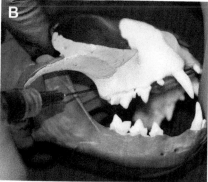

Fig. 4. Extraoral maxillary nerve block. (*A*) Dog. (*B*) Cat. © 2019 Ana C. Castejón-González and Alexander M. Reiter.

lip. Once injected, apply finger pressure for a few seconds to avoid reflux of the local anesthetic solution (see **Fig. 3**).

Inferior Alveolar Nerve Block

The inferior alveolar nerve block is used for procedures of the mandibular body, its teeth, surrounding oral mucosa, and lower lip. There is collateral innervation to the skin and the periosteum of the mandible by both the facial and trigeminal nerves; therefore, complete desensitization of the mandible and intermandibular tissues cannot be accomplished even with bilateral inferior alveolar nerve blocks.[17,18] The inferior alveolar nerve enters the mandibular canal through the mandibular foramen, which is located medially at the ventral aspect of the mandibular ramus, about halfway between the last molar tooth and the angular process of the mandible. The foramen and the neurovascular bundle before entering the mandibular canal can be palpated intraorally in many patients, but it might be difficult to do so in cats and small dogs. The local anesthetic solution is deposited next to the mandibular foramen but not into the mandibular canal.[16]

- Intraoral approach
  - The landmarks for this approach are the last molar tooth, the angular process of the mandible, and the mandibular foramen.
  - The thumb of the nondominant hand is placed caudal to the last molar tooth and the index finger over the angular process of the mandible to estimate the distance between these 2 landmarks.
  - Using the dominant hand, the needle penetrates the oral mucosa linguodistal to the last molar tooth. The angle between the needle and the dorsal margin of the mandible should be 20° to 25°.
  - The needle is advanced caudally as close to the mandible as possible, slightly more than half of the distance between the index finger and the thumb. It should not be advanced medially toward the tongue so as to avoid inadvertent blockade of the lingual nerve (**Fig. 5**).
- Extraoral approach
  - The landmarks for this approach are an unnamed notch (palpable in the dog but barely present in the cat) at the ventral margin of the mandibular ramus, the last molar tooth, and the angular process.

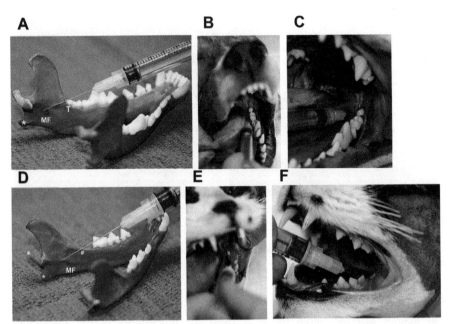

Fig. 5. Intraoral inferior alveolar nerve block. (*A*) The needle is advanced between the last molar tooth (T) toward the angular process of the mandibular ramus (*asterisk*) up to the mandibular foramen (MF) in a dog. (*B*) Insertion of the needle in the lingual mucosa medial to the mandible. The needle is oriented laterally toward the bone. (*C*) Approximate angle between the needle and the mandible. (*D*) The needle is advanced from the end of the mandibular body (*hash mark*) toward the angular process of the mandibular ramus (*asterisk*) up to the MF in a cat. (*E*) Insertion of the needle in the mucosa caudal and lingual to the mandibular first molar tooth. Do not traumatize the linguomolar salivary gland (S). (*F*) Approximate angle between the needle and the mandible. © 2019 Ana C. Castejón-González and Alexander M. Reiter.

- The mandibular foramen is located dorsal to the unnamed notch about halfway along a line drawn between the last molar tooth and angular process of the mandible.
- The needle is inserted through the skin ventromedial to the mandible at the level of the unnamed notch.
- The needle is advanced along the medial aspect of the ramus of the mandible in a dorsocaudal direction (**Fig. 6**).
- In cats, the unnamed notch is very subtle. Some authors draw a line from the lateral canthus of the eye up to the facial notch to decide where the needle should penetrate the skin.[6]

Middle Mental Nerve Block

The anesthetic drug is deposited at the level of the middle mental foramen usually without advancing the needle into the mandibular canal. In medium-sized and large dogs, the foramen is large enough to allow for slight advancement of the needle into the canal. If the drug is deposited at the level of the middle mental foramen, the rostral lower lip and oral mucosa on that side are desensitized. Blockade of the alveolar branches that supply the incisor, canine, and most rostral premolar teeth and surrounding tissues only occurs if the anesthetic solution is placed into the mandibular

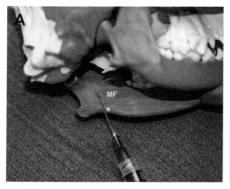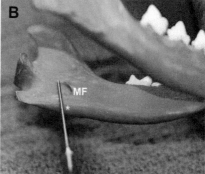

Fig. 6. Extraoral inferior alveolar nerve block. (*A*) Dog. (*B*) Cat. The needle is advanced from the unnamed notch (*asterisk*) caudally toward the mandibular foramen (MF). The solution is placed caudal and dorsal to the MF in the area where the nerve runs before it enters the canal. © 2019 Ana C. Castejón-González and Alexander M. Reiter.

canal. An experimental study conducted in dogs showed that most tissues evaluated (mucogingival junction, mucocutaneous junction, and mandibular teeth) still expressed sensitivity after a middle mental nerve block even though the local anesthetic solution was placed into the mandibular canal.[19] The authors use the middle mental nerve block only for small procedures in the rostral lower lip (eg, biopsies, repair of small lacerations). For more involved procedures (eg, root canal therapy, repair of lower lip avulsion or mandibular symphysial separation, tooth extractions, mandibulectomy), the inferior alveolar nerve block is preferred.

- The needle is inserted in the oral mucosa rostral to the lip frenulum.
- The needle is advanced in a ventrocaudal direction toward the middle mental foramen. In dogs, the middle mental foramen can be palpated ventral to the mesial root of the second premolar tooth. In cats, the middle mental foramen is located slightly caudal to the apex of the canine tooth (**Fig. 7**).
- In medium-sized and large dogs, the needle can be advanced slightly into the mandibular canal.

Major Palatine Nerve Block

The blockade of the major palatine nerve desensitizes the ipsilateral soft tissue and bone of the hard palate rostral to the block. Introduction of the needle into the palatine canal is not recommended so as to avoid injury of the major palatine artery and nerve. The major palatine foramen cannot be palpated. It is located halfway between the midline of the palate and the distal root of the maxillary fourth premolar tooth in most dogs. In cats and brachycephalic dogs, the foramen is located slightly more rostrally between the midline of the palate and the mesial roots of the maxillary fourth premolar tooth.[3,9,16]

- The needle should penetrate the oral mucosa 2 to 3 palatine rugae rostral to the major palatine foramen.
- The needle is advanced caudally just a few millimeters rostral to the foramen (**Fig. 8**).
- Following injection, a small bulge may be visible and palpable in the hard palate mucosa. Injection of an excessive volume of local anesthetic solution can cause pressure ischemia of the oral mucosa.

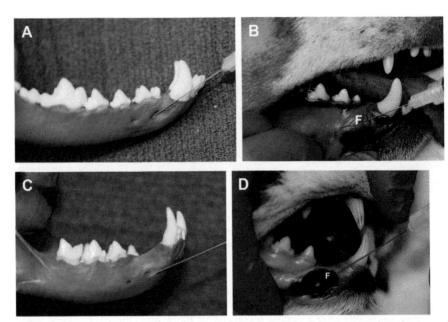

Fig. 7. Middle mental nerve block. (*A*) The middle mental foramen is ventral to the second premolar tooth in the dog. (*B*) Insertion of the needle occurs rostral to the lip frenulum (F). (*C*) The middle mental foramen is located at the level of the apex of the canine tooth in the cat. The needle is placed rostral to the foramen. (*D*) Insertion of the needle occurs rostral to the lip frenulum (F). © 2019 Ana C. Castejón-González and Alexander M. Reiter.

REGIONAL ANESTHESIA OF THE EYE

The main regional blocks are the retrobulbar and peribulbar nerve blocks.

Neuroanatomy

The innervation of the eye is provided by the optic, oculomotor, and trochlear nerves, the ophthalmic and maxillary branches of the trigeminal nerve, the abducens nerve, and the auriculopalpebral branch of the facial nerve. The oculomotor, trochlear, ophthalmic, abducens, and facial nerves deliver motor innervation to the eye and eyelids. The ophthalmic nerve is responsible for most of the sensory innervation of the eye and orbit along with the zygomatic nerve that arises from the maxillary nerve.[12,17,24]

Retrobulbar Block

The retrobulbar block desensitizes the oculomotor, trochlear, ophthalmic, and abducens nerves, and the ciliary ganglion. The objective is to place the local anesthetic into to the orbital apex inside the extraocular muscle cone. This technique is useful for adjuvant analgesia in enucleation, evisceration, and intraocular surgery. If the block is successful, it causes centralization of the eye, mild exophthalmos, and mydriasis.[8,12,24,25]

- Inferior-temporal palpebral (ITP) approach[10,12,25]
  - A 22-gauge spinal needle or 1.5-inch hypodermic needle is manually curved by about 10° to 20° (**Fig. 9**).
  - The needle is inserted between the lateral and middle third of the lower eyelid through the skin or conjunctiva (**Fig. 10**).

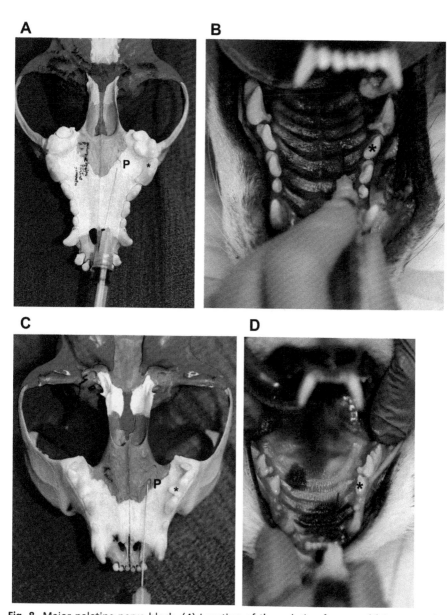

Fig. 8. Major palatine nerve block. (*A*) Location of the palatine foramen (P) between the midline of the palate and the distal root of the maxillary fourth premolar tooth (*asterisk*) in a dog. (*B*) Insertion of the needle in the palatal mucosa at the level of the maxillary third premolar tooth (*asterisk*). (*C*) The palatine foramen (P) in the cat is located more rostral compared with the dog, at the level of the mesial roots of the maxillary fourth premolar tooth (*asterisk*). (*D*) Insertion of the needle in the mucosa at the level of the maxillary third premolar tooth (asterisk). © 2019 Ana C. Castejón-González and Alexander M. Reiter.

- The needle is initially advanced toward the retrobulbar area along the floor of the orbit until the orbital fascia is perforated (a popping sensation may be noted in dogs), then the needle is oriented dorsonasally and advanced 1 to 2 cm toward the apex of the orbit.
- The anesthetic solution should be injected slowly.

- Dorsomedial approach

  This approach is preferred in cats because injection by the ITP retrobulbar technique does not result in an adequate distribution of the anesthetic solution in the retrobulbar area.[26] The needle is inserted transcutaneously between the medial and middle third of the upper eyelid and then advanced toward the retrobulbar space (see **Fig. 10**). Perforation of the orbital fascia is not noted.[27]

- Perimandibular approach[10,12]

  - A straight needle should penetrate the skin ventral to the zygomatic arch at the level of the lateral canthus of the eye (see **Fig. 10**).
  - The needle is advanced medially, dorsally, and caudally to reach the retrobulbar space.

- Lateral canthus approach[12]

  - A straight needle is inserted transconjunctivally at the lateral canthus of the eye (see **Fig. 10**).
  - The needle is oriented in a ventromedial direction toward the retrobulbar space.

- Supratemporal approach[28]

  This approach has only been described in cadavers. The authors have suggested that it is technically easier to perform than the ITP technique.[28]

  - A straight needle is inserted in the skin caudal to the orbital ligament and dorsal to the zygomatic arch (see **Fig. 10**).
  - The needle is oriented medioventrally at an angle of 80° to 90° until the extraocular muscles are perforated.

- Combined superior-inferior peribulbar approach[10,12,24]

  - This approach needs 2 injection points, one dorsal and another ventral to the globe. The dorsal point of injection is at the upper eyelid and the ventral point of injection at the lower eyelid, both midway between the lateral and medial canthi of the eye (see **Fig. 10**).
  - The needle is advanced between the globe and the orbital rim up to the retrobulbar area.

Three of the aforementioned techniques were compared in dogs.[10] The ITP approach showed better distribution of the injected latex and contrast material intraconally than the perimandibular technique or the combined superior-inferior peribulbar technique, as well as absence of complications. Based on these results, the ITP approach is preferred in dogs and the dorsomedial approach is preferred in cats.[10,26]

A   **B**

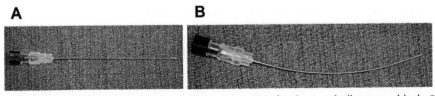

Fig. 9. (*A*) Spinal needle. (*B*) Spinal needle bent about 20° for the retrobulbar nerve block. © 2019 Ana C. Castejón-González and Alexander M. Reiter.

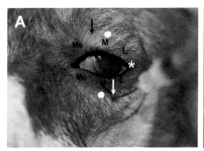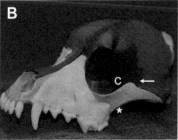

Fig. 10. Points of injection for the retrobulbar nerve block. (*A*) The needle is inserted in the lower eyelid between the lateral (L) and middle (M) thirds of the eyelid in the inferior-temporal-palpebral approach (*white arrow*). The 2 white dots indicate the insertion points of the needles for the combined superior-inferior approach. The lateral canthus approach is marked with an asterisk. The needle is inserted between the medial (Me) and middle (M) thirds of the upper eyelid for the dorsomedial technique (*black arrow*). (*B*) Representation of the points of injection for the perimandibular (*asterisk*) and the supratemporal (*arrow*) approaches. The needle should be oriented toward the retrobulbar area, inside the extraocular muscles cone (C). © 2019 Ana C. Castejón-González and Alexander M. Reiter.

Peribulbar Block

The peribulbar block desensitizes the globe and the periocular tissues including the eyelids.[12] If the anesthetic solution diffuses intraconally, it can also decrease the sensitivity of the cornea.[27,29] The volume of local anesthetic used for this technique is larger in comparison with the retrobulbar technique, which might elevate intraocular pressure and increase the risk of toxicity. The local anesthetic can be diluted with saline to increase the volume. Its use in eyes with glaucoma or at risk of rupture is contraindicated unless they are scheduled for enucleation. The local anesthetic is placed outside of the extraocular muscle cone.[12,24]

- The local anesthetic solution is injected subconjunctivally dorsal, lateral, ventral, and medial to the globe.[12]
- A 2-points injection technique has been described for dogs and cats. The full length of a ⅝- to 1-inch 25-gauge needle is inserted through the upper eyelid in a dorsomedial location, and another needle in a ventrolateral location through the lower eyelid. The needles are advanced into the orbit between the extraocular muscles and the bone.[25]
- In cats, a 1-point technique also was described by injecting the anesthetic solution in a dorsomedial location in the upper eyelid.[26,27]

In studies comparing the retrobulbar and peribulbar techniques in dogs and cats, the peribulbar technique was able to diffuse inside the extraocular muscular cone and cause anesthesia of the periorbital tissues and the cornea.[25,27]

REGIONAL ANESTHESIA OF THE EAR

The 2 nerve blocks that are used together to provide some pain relief in ear surgery are the great auricular nerve block and auriculotemporal nerve block.[30,31]

Neuroanatomy

The innervation of the ear is complex. The cutaneous innervation is supplied by branches of second cervical, trigeminal, and facial nerves. The dorsal branch (occipitoauricular) and one of the ventral branches (great auricular nerve) of the second cervical nerve supply the caudal and lateral aspects of the pinna, but these areas overlap with the area of innervation of the trigeminal and facial nerves. The auriculotemporal nerve, a branch of the mandibular nerve, supplies sensory innervation to the medioventral part of the pinna and the tympanic membrane.[32] Therefore, complete desensitization of the ear is not possible, and other adjuvant methods of pain control are necessary for surgical procedures of the ear.

Great Auricular Nerve Block

- The nerve is located relatively superficial, ventral to the wing of the atlas and caudal to the tympanic bulla.[30,31]
- The needle is inserted in the skin ventral to the atlas and caudal to the ear canal.
- The needle is advanced ventral and cranial into the subcutaneous tissue.
- The solution is injected caudal to the vertical ear canal.

A cadaveric study suggested the injection in 3 points to cover the whole length of the transverse process of the atlas, with the needle oriented toward the jugular groove.[33] This approach can potentially block both branches of the second cervical nerve.

Auriculotemporal Nerve Block

- The needle is inserted in the skin between the rostral aspect of the ear canal and the zygomatic arch.[30,31]
- The needle is advanced half of the distance between the skin and the bone.

INFILTRATION ANESTHESIA

The local anesthetic is injected around the planned incision to desensitize the terminal nerve endings.[3] Lidocaine and bupivacaine are the most frequently used local anesthetic drugs, but a slow-release form of bupivacaine (bupivacaine liposome injectable suspension) has recently been introduced to the veterinary community. Bupivacaine liposome injectable suspension provides pain relief for up to 72 hours[34]; however, desensitization and numbness of the face for such a long time might not be necessary depending on the procedure or pain level. Inadvertent desensitization of the tongue caused by infiltration of the bupivacaine liposome injectable suspension and subsequent blockade of the lingual nerve likely causes lingual injury from teeth biting into the tongue. Infiltration of the surgical site with bupivacaine liposome injectable suspension was used off-label in mandibulectomy and maxillectomy procedures for postoperative pain control, with good results. It has also potential application for nerve blocks, but currently there is not enough published information about its application in oral and maxillofacial surgery.[34] Infiltration of a local anesthetic in the eyelids is useful after enucleation or eyelid surgery or as an adjunct to retrobulbar anesthesia. Preoperative infiltration might cause deformation of the eyelids and interfere with the surgical procedure unless a small volume of anesthetic solution is injected.[12] The injection is performed along the skin and subcutaneous tissue as the needle is slowly withdrawn. The infiltration can also be used after completion of a surgical procedure for immediate postoperative pain control.[12]

SPLASH BLOCK (WOUND IRRIGATION)

This technique consists of dropping the local anesthetic solution into the open wound before closure of the surgical area.[35] Vasoconstrictors can be mixed with the local anesthetic to decrease diffuse bleeding and increase the duration of the anesthetic

Table 4
(continued)

Complication	Nerve Block	Comments
Infection	All locoregional techniques	Rinse the mouth with chlorhexidine 0.12% before giving any intraoral nerve block; prepare aseptically the area of cutaneous injection; use aseptic techniques
Delayed healing and wound dehiscence	Infiltration techniques	Do not infiltrate more than 5 mL per eye[12]
Oculocardiac reflex	Locoregional anesthesia of the eye, maxillary nerve block (transorbital approach)	Regional anesthesia reduces the oculocardiac reflex, but it can also induce it, causing bradycardia and asystole. Trigeminocardiac reflex can also occur by manipulation, such as stretching of nerves of the oral cavity
Intravascular injection	Regional nerve blocks, infiltration	If lidocaine is administered intravascularly, the dose used for a nerve block is usually not enough to cause signs of systemic toxicity; there is a higher risk of having hypotension or cardiovascular complications if bupivacaine is used; aspirate before injecting; rapid absorption with hypotension can also occur in the absence of intravascular injection

*from Refs.[21,36–43]

.[9] A mixture of 0.25 mL of phenylephrine 1% and 50 mL of lidocaine 2% is ...ely applied by the authors into the nasal cavity after maxillectomy procedures ...alate defect repairs. Half the volume is applied directly into the nasal cavity ...e wound closure and the other half through the ipsilateral nostril (or both nostrils ...ding on the procedure performed) after wound closure. The total dose of the ...re is 0.1 to 0.2 mL/kg in dogs and 0.05 to 0.1 mL/kg in cats.[35] In ocular surgery, ...sh block of the orbit with the local anesthetic alone or impregnated in an absorb-...elatin hemostatic sponge can be used after enucleation or evisceration.[11,36] The ...anesthetic (bupivacaine, ropivacaine) is left in the wound from 30 seconds to ...ttes before closing it.

...LICATIONS

...act complication rate of locoregional anesthesia of the head in dogs and cats is ...wn. Although many complications are possible, in the authors' experience they ... happen frequently. Use of smaller needles, aspiration before injection, staying ... the maximum safe dose, minimizing the injected volume, and knowing the

Table 4
Complications associated with locoregional anesthesia of the head

Complication	Nerve Block	Comments
Hematoma	Potential complication with all nerve blocks	Retrobulbar he (maxillary ne retrobulbar cause exoph ptosis[39]
Nerve damage	Potential complication with all nerve blocks	Can cause dec of the area, neuropathi needles cau neurovascu not insert t canals (ie, mandibula the menta dogs and
Vision loss	Retrobulbar anesthesia, maxillary nerve block	Damage of penetrati globe.[21,3] might be
Exophthalmos	Retrobulbar nerve block, maxillary nerve block	Caused by injected or hema tears in period
Corneal ulcers	Locoregional anesthesia of the eye	Decreased ability effect permar exopht tears u functi produ
Uveitis	Locoregional anesthesia of the eye, maxillary block	Early op evalua
Conjunctival hyperemia	Peribulbar and retrobulbar block	Usually
Intrathecal administration	Retrobulbar nerve block	The op cove shea anes repc caus
Lingual trauma	Inferior alveolar nerve block	By usi diff ner the kee mc th se

anatomy of the target area help to avoid complications.[3,9] Complications derived from administration of local anesthetics are listed in **Table 4**.[21,36–43] The retrobulbar block may have more complications than the periocular or splash block, in particular when the intraconal injection technique is used.[11,36] **Box 1** shows a practical check list to prevent complications.

SUMMARY

Locoregional anesthesia plays an important role in multimodal analgesic protocols. It is considered safe as long as precautions are taken before and during administration of the anesthetic solution. Cadaver practice will enable the veterinarian to become more comfortable and efficient with the various techniques. Locoregional anesthesia is recommended for many surgical procedures of the oral cavity, eye, and ear.

REFERENCES

1. Muir W, Berry J, Merton Boothe D, et al. Opioid-sparing pain therapy in animals: working task force. Conifer (CO): American College of Veterinary Anesthesia and Analgesia; 2018. Available at: http://www.acvaa.org. Accessed February 20, 2019.
2. Aguiar J, Chebroux A, Martinez-Taboada F, et al. Analgesic effects of maxillary and inferior alveolar nerve blocks in cats undergoing dental extractions. J Feline Med Surg 2015;17:110–6.
3. Gracis M. The oral cavity. In: Matt R, Campoy L, editors. Small animal regional anesthesia and analgesia. Ames (IA): Wiley-Blackwell; 2013. p. 131–55.
4. Fizzano KM, Claude AK, Kuo L, et al. Evaluation of a modified infraorbital approach for a maxillary nerve block for rhinoscopy with nasal biopsy of dogs. Am J Vet Res 2017;78:1025–35.
5. Snyder CJ, Snyder LB. Effect of mepivacaine in an infraorbital nerve block on minimum alveolar concentration of isoflurane in clinically normal anesthetized dogs undergoing a modified form of dental dolorimetry. J Am Vet Med Assoc 2013;242:199–204.
6. Beckman B. Anesthesia and pain management for small animals. Vet Clin North Am Small Anim Pract 2013;43:669–88.
7. Buback JL, Boothe HW, Carroll GL, et al. Comparison of three methods for relief of pain after ear canal ablation in dogs. Vet Surg 1996;25:380–5.
8. Myrna KE, Bentley E, Smith LJ. Effectiveness of injection of local anesthetic into the retrobulbar space for postoperative analgesia following eye enucleation in dog. J Am Vet Med Assoc 2010;237:174–7.
9. Johnston N, Larenza Menzies MP. Anaesthetic and analgesic considerations in dentistry and oral surgery. In: Reiter AM, Gracis M, editors. BSAVA manual of canine and feline dentistry and oral surgery. 4th edition. Gloucester (England): BSAVA; 2018. p. 119–36.
10. Accola PJ, Bentley E, Smith LJ, et al. Development of a retrobulbar injection technique for ocular surgery and analgesia in dogs. J Am Vet Med Assoc 2006;229:220–5.
11. Chow DWY, Wong MY, Westermeyer H. Comparison of two bupivacaine delivery methods to control postoperative pain after enucleation in dogs. Vet Ophthalmol 2015;18:422–8.
12. Giuliano EA, Walsh KP. The eye. In: Matt R, Campoy L, editors. Small animal regional anesthesia and analgesia. Ames (IA): Wiley-Blackwell; 2013. p. 115–30.

13. Pascoe PJ. The effects of lidocaine or a lidocaine-bupivacaine mixture administered into the infraorbital canal in dogs. Am J Vet Res 2016;77:682–7.
14. Rochette J. Regional anesthesia and analgesia for oral and dental procedures. Vet Clin North Am Small Anim Pract 2005;35:1041–58.
15. Milella L, Gurney M. Dental and oral surgery. In: Duke-Novakovski T, de Vries M, Seymour C, editors. Canine and feline anaesthesia and analgesia. 3rd edition. Gloucester (England): BSAVA; 2016. p. 272–82.
16. Lantz GC. Regional anesthesia for dentistry and oral surgery. J Vet Dent 2003;20:181–6.
17. Evans H, Lahunta A. Cranial nerves. In: Evans HE, de Lahunta A, editors. Miller's anatomy of the dog. St. Louis (MO): Saunders; 2013. p. 708–30.
18. Cremer J, Sum SO, Braun C, et al. Assessment of maxillary and infraorbital nerve blockade for rhinoscopy in sevoflurane anesthetized dog. Vet Anaesth Analg 2013;40:432–9.
19. Krug W, Losey J. Area of desensitization following mental nerve block in dogs. J Vet Dent 2011;28:146–50.
20. Viscasillas J, Seymour CJ, Brodbelt DC. A cadaver study comparing two approaches for performing maxillary nerve block in dogs. Vet Anaesth Analg 2013;40:212–9.
21. Perry R, Moore D, Scurrell E. Globe penetration in a cat following maxillary nerve block for dental surgery. J Feline Med Surg 2015;17:66–72.
22. Gracis M, Harvey CE. Radiographic study of the maxillary canine tooth in four mesaticephalic cats. J Vet Dent 1999;16:115–8.
23. Langton SD, Walker JJA. A transorbital approach to the maxillary nerve block in dogs: a cadaver study. Vet Anaesth Analg 2017;44:173–7.
24. Shilo Benjamini Y. A review of ophthalmic local and regional anesthesia in dogs and cats. Vet Anaesth Analg 2019;46:14–27.
25. Shilo-Benjamini Y, Pascoe PJ, Wisner ER, et al. A comparison of retrobulbar and two peribulbar regional anesthetic techniques in dog cadavers. Vet Anaesth Analg 2017;44:925–32.
26. Shilo- Benjamini Y, Pascoe PJ, Maggs DJ, et al. Retrobulbar and peribulbar regional techniques in cats: a preliminary study in cadavers. Vet Anaesth Analg 2013;40:623–31.
27. Shilo- Benjamini Y, Pascoe PJ, Maggs DJ, et al. Comparison of peribulbar and retrobulbar regional anesthesia with bupivacaine in cats. Am J Vet Res 2014;75:1029–39.
28. Chiavaccini L, Micieli F, Meomartino L, et al. A novel supra-temporal approach to retrobulbar anesthesia in dogs: preliminary study in cadavers. Vet J 2017;223:68–70.
29. Shilo-Benjamini Y, Pascoe PJ, Maggs DJ, et al. Retrobulbar vs peribulbar regional anesthesia techniques using bupivacaine in dogs. Vet Ophthalmol 2018. https://doi.org/10.1111/vop.12579.
30. Duke-Novakovski T. Pain management II: local and regional anesthetic techniques. In: Duke-Novakovski T, de Vries M, Seymour C, editors. Canine and feline anaesthesia and analgesia. 3rd edition. Gloucester (England): BSAVA; 2016. p. 143–58.
31. Taboada-Martinez F. Blocks of the head. In: Lerche P, Aarnes TK, Covey-Crump G, et al, editors. Handbook of small animal regional anesthesia and analgesia techniques. Oxford: Wiley Blackwell; 2016. p. 37–52.
32. Evans H, Lahunta A. Spinal nerves. In: Evans HE, de Lahunta A, editors. Miller's anatomy of the dog. St. Louis (MO): Saunders; 2013. p. 611–57.

33. Stathopoulou TR, Pinelas R, Ter Haar G, et al. Description of a new approach for great auricular and auriculotemporal nerve blocks: a cadaveric study in foxes and dogs. Vet Med Sci 2018;4:91–7.
34. Lascelles BD, Shaw KK. An extended release local anaesthetic: potential for future use in veterinary surgical patients? Vet Med Sci 2016;2:229–38.
35. Reiter AM. Equipment for oral surgery in small animal practice. Vet Clin North Am Small Anim Pract 2013;43:587–608.
36. Ploog CL, Swinger RL, Spade J, et al. Use of lidocaine-bupivacaine-infused absorbable gelatin hemostatic sponges versus lidocaine-bupivacaine retrobulbar injections for postoperative analgesia following eye enucleation in dogs. J Am Vet Med Assoc 2014;244:57–62.
37. Alessio TL, Krieger EM. Transient unilateral vision loss in a dog following inadvertent intravitreal injection of bupivacaine during a dental procedure. J Am Vet Med Assoc 2015;246:990993.
38. Aprea F, Vettorato E, Corletto F. Severe cardiovascular depression in a cat following a mandibular nerve block with bupivacaine. Vet Anaesth Analg 2011; 38:614–8.
39. Loughran CM, Raisis AL, Hatijema G, et al. Unilateral retrobulbar hematoma following maxillary nerve block in a dog. J Vet Emerg Crit Care (San Antonio) 2016;26:815–8.
40. Snyder LB, Snyder CJ, Hetzel S. Effects of buprenorphine added to bupivacaine infraorbital nerve blocks on isoflurane minimum alveolar concentration using a model for acute dental/oral surgical pain in dogs. J Vet Dent 2016;33:90–6.
41. Volk HA, Bayley KD, Fiani N, et al. Ophthalmic complications following ocular penetration during routine dentistry in 13 cats. N Z Vet J 2019;67:46–51.
42. Oliver JA, Bradbrook CA. Suspect brainstem anesthesia following retrobulbar block in a cat. Vet Ophthalmol 2013;16:225–8.
43. Vezina-Audette R, Benedicenti L, Castejon-Gonzalez A, et al. Anesthesia case of the month: Recurrent asystole and severe bradycardia during surgical repair of cleft palate in a dog. J Am Vet Med Assoc 2017;250:1104–6.

Locoregional Anesthesia of the Thoracic Limbs and Thorax in Small Animals

Diego A. Portela, MV, PhD[a],*, Marta Romano, DVM, MSc, PhD[a],
Pablo E. Otero, MV, PhD[b]

KEYWORDS

- Regional anesthesia • Brachial plexus block • Subscalene • RUMM block
- Thoracic paravertebral block • Erector spinae plane block • Small animals

KEY POINTS

- Ultrasound guidance and nerve stimulation facilitate the execution of nerve blocks of the thoracic limb and thorax.
- The brachial plexus can be blocked using a subscalene or axillary approach to provide analgesia to the entire thoracic limb or distal to the mid-humerus, respectively.
- Proximal and distal radial, ulnar, median and musculocutaneous nerve blocks are adequate alternatives to the brachial plexus block.
- Intercostal and thoracic paravertebral nerve blocks may be used to provide somatic and both somatic and visceral thoracic analgesia, respectively.
- Erector spinae plane block is a novel technique used to desensitize the epaxial musculature and the dorsal aspect of the vertebral column.

INTRODUCTION

Research studies focusing on the development of novel regional anesthesia techniques for animals have become more common in the last 2 decades. The incorporation of objective methods to assess the position of the needle in relationship to the nerve, such as nerve stimulation (NS) and ultrasound (US) guidance, have contributed to increasing the accuracy and success rate of nerve blocks while possibly reducing the risks of complications associated with blind techniques.[1,2]

Disclosure Statement: The authors do not have any conflict of interest to write this article.
[a] Anesthesiology and Pain Management, Department of Comparative, Diagnostic, and Population Medicine, College of Veterinary Medicine, University of Florida, 2015 Southwest 16th Avenue, PO Box 100123, Gainesville, FL 32610-0136, USA; [b] Anesthesiology and Pain Management Department, Facultad de Ciencias Veterinarias, Universidad de Buenos Aires, Avenida Chorroarín 280 (C1427CWO), Buenos Aires, Argentina
* Corresponding author.
E-mail address: dportela@ufl.edu

The ongoing opioid shortage crisis as well as an increased awareness of the possible benefits and decreased incidence of side effects when regional anesthesia is used has resulted in increased interest in the development of novel techniques aimed at desensitizing selected areas of the body.[3,4] When performed correctly, these regional anesthesia techniques can either constitute an alternative to opioid and other systemic analgesic use, or have a significant opioid-sparing effect.[5,6] Moreover, by blocking input to the central nervous system, regional anesthesia can help to prevent the development of pathologic pain conditions.[7] Although most of the described regional anesthesia techniques for animals have focused on the thoracic and pelvic limbs, multiple techniques to desensitize different areas of the trunk have been published in the recent years.[8,9] This article focuses on reviewing the current literature and describing some of the published regional anesthesia techniques for the thoracic limb and thorax in small animal patients.

GENERAL CONSIDERATIONS IN PERFORMING LOCOREGIONAL ANESTHESIA TECHNIQUES

The use of NS and US guidance has been introduced in veterinary medicine to decrease the subjectivity of blind nerve blocks, improve accuracy, and decrease the occurrence of complications. Familiarity with the appropriate equipment to perform regional anesthesia and with the techniques of nerve location are essential to reduce the risks of potential complications, such as nerve damage, hematoma formation, and intravascular injection (**Fig. 1**). Proper aseptic technique through appropriate clipping, skin preparation, and the use of sterile materials should be observed when performing nerve blocks. Extravascular positioning of the tip of the needle should always be confirmed by the aspiration test before injecting a local anesthetic (see **Fig. 1**). High resistance ($\geq$15 psi) or nociceptive reaction to injection could indicate that the needle tip is positioned intraneurally.[10] If this occurs, the injection should be discontinued immediately and the needle repositioned.

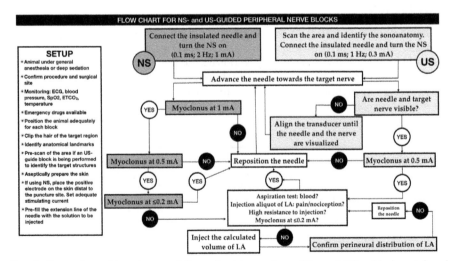

Fig. 1. General considerations and flow chart to perform NS- and US-guided peripheral nerve blocks. ECG, electraocardiogram; ETCO$_2$, end-tital carbon dioxide; LA, local anesthetic; SpO$_2$, peripheral capillary oxygen saturation.

When NS is used for nerve location, the correct muscular response should be elicited with an electrical current between 0.3 and 0.5 mA. A positive myoclonus with 0.2 mA or less may indicate that the tip of the needle is positioned intraneurally; therefore, the needle must be repositioned before injecting. US guidance with continuous visualization of the tip of the needle decreases the risks of accidental intraneural or intravascular injection. The needle should not be advanced until its tip is visualized.

Vigilant cardiovascular monitoring should be performed in patients receiving a nerve block to promptly detect any signs of local anesthetic toxicity and establish appropriate treatment.

For most of the techniques described in this article, long-acting local anesthetics, such as bupivacaine or ropivacaine 0.5% are recommended. Exceeding the maximum recommended doses for each species should be avoided to reduce the risks of systemic toxicity. If large volumes of local anesthetic are necessary, their concentration may be decreased (ie, $\leq$0.25%) to avoid exceeding the recommended doses. Low concentrations of long-acting local anesthetics are effective at providing sensory blockade, while limiting the duration and intensity of the motor blockade.

Brachial Plexus Block: Subscalene Approach

The brachial plexus block through a subscalene approach aims to block the primary ventral branches of C6, C7, C8, and T1 spinal nerves as they run in the caudoventral aspect of the neck, between the scalenus ventralis and the longus colli muscles, before reaching the axillary space.[11] A preliminary cadaveric study showed that when 2 volumes of dye (0.3 and 0.4 mL/kg) were injected using an US-guided approach, C7, C8, T1, and the phrenic nerve were consistently stained with both volumes, whereas C6 was only stained when the higher volume was used.[11] Neither of the volumes used in this study were associated with epidural, intrapleural, or mediastinal distribution of the dye solution. One clinical report evaluating the diaphragmatic function via M-mode ultrasonography in dogs administered a subscalene brachial plexus block for forelimb surgery revealed that the diaphragmatic movement was impaired in all animals 20 minutes after the injection of 0.3 mL/kg of bupivacaine 0.5%.[12]

There are no clinical studies evaluating the efficacy of this technique. However, based on the authors' experience, this approach can be used for procedures involving the proximal third of the forelimb, including scapulohumeral joint surgeries. This block may also be used in animals undergoing thoracic limb amputations. However, because the proximal scapular area is innervated by the dorsal rami of the spinal nerves and the accessory nerve, additional analgesia should be planned to complement the subscalene brachial plexus block in animals undergoing forelimb amputation with scapulectomy.

Relevant anatomy

The brachial plexus is formed by the primary ventral rami of the spinal nerves C6, C7, C8, and T1, with occasional contribution from C5 and T2.[13] As the ventral rami of the spinal nerves leave the intervertebral foramen, they run in a caudolateral direction aligned in the intermuscular plane formed by the scalenus ventralis and the longus colli muscles, surrounded by the deep fascia of the neck laterally and the prevertebral fascia medially (**Fig. 2**D).

The phrenic nerve runs along the ventral margin of the scalenus muscle, medially to the brachial plexus, in the same interfascial compartment.[14] The ventral rami of C6, C7, C8, and T1 provide sensory innervation to the shoulder, brachium, antebrachium, and manus (**Fig. 2**B). The skin of the caudomedial aspect of the arm, from the axilla to

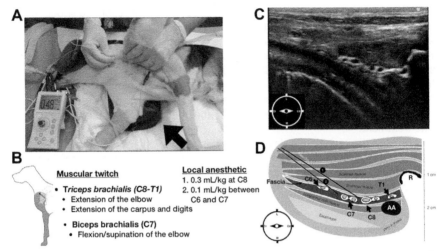

Fig. 2. US-guided subscalene brachial plexus block. (*A*) Dog and transducer position for US-guided technique. A rolled towel or a pillow (*black arrow*) is positioned under the dependent shoulder to displace the upper scapula caudally and expose the brachial plexus. (*B*) Desensitized anatomical area. (*C*) US image of the brachial plexus through a subscalene approach. (*D*) Schematic representation of (*C*): needle positioned for injecting the local anesthetic at T8 (1) and between C6 and C7 (2). AA, axillary artery; Cd, caudal; Cr, cranial; L, lateral; M, medial.

the elbow, is innervated by the intercostobrachial nerve, which is not blocked when performing this technique.

Ultrasound-guided technique
Owing to the proximity of the brachial plexus to the thoracic inlet, this technique should be performed under direct US visualization to minimize the risk of accidental intrathoracic puncture. NS can be used in association to US guidance to confirm correct needle positioning.

Technique
- Position the patient in lateral recumbency with the limb to be blocked uppermost and in a neutral position. Place a round cushion under the dependent shoulder to achieve caudal displacement of the upper scapula and extension of the neck (**Fig. 2**A).
- Position the US transducer parallel to the longitudinal axis of the scalenus muscle, cranial to the first rib and above the costochondral joint, with the marker oriented cranially.
- Slide the transducer caudally while displacing the scapula, until the first rib can be visualized (**Fig. 2**C), then move the transducer dorsally until the C6, C7, C8, and T1 nerve roots can be visualized medially to the belly of the scalenus muscle, under the deep fascia of the neck. Tilt the transducer to obtain a clear image of the nerves and of the deep fascia of the neck and identify the axillary artery, located caudally and medially to T1.
- Sonoanatomy of the brachial plexus in the subscalene space (see **Fig. 2**C, D):
  - The first rib is visualized as a hyperechoic structure projecting an acoustic shadow.

- The nerves forming the brachial plexus are located cranially to the first rib and can be visualized as round structures aligned between the deep fascia of the neck and the prevertebral fascia.
  - The axillary artery is located medially to the nerve complex.
- Introduce a 21G insulated needle ventral to the transverse prosses of the sixth cervical vertebra, cranial and in-plane to the transducer (see **Fig. 2**A). The authors recommend using 50-mm needles for cats and dogs smaller than 5 kg and, 75 to 100 mm for medium and large size dogs.
- Set the NS to 0.3 mA, 1 Hz, and 0.1 ms. When the tip of the needle is in proximity to one of the target nerves, the electrical current on the NS should be increased to 0.5 mA to confirm the correct muscular response. Depending on which nerves are being stimulated, one of the following muscular responses can be elicited:
  - C6: adduction and extension of the shoulder.
  - C7: flexion of the elbow and shoulder.
  - C8 to T1: extension of the elbow and extension or flexion of the carpal joint and digits.
- Advance the needle toward the caudal aspect of C7, piercing the deep fascia of the neck.
- After confirming the extravascular positioning of the tip of the needle, 0.4 mL/kg of local anesthetic should be injected.
  - Three-quarters of the total calculated volume (0.3 mL/kg) should be injected on the caudal aspect of C7. The needle should then be withdrawn slightly and redirected cranially to C7, where the rest of the local anesthetic solution (0.1 mL/kg) should be deposited.

Potential complications

Diaphragmatic hemiparesis has been reported after a subscalene brachial plexus block owing to unilateral phrenic blockade.[12] Although specific studies are lacking, several complications may occur in association to this technique, owing to the anatomy of the brachial plexus and surrounding structures at this level, including:

- Vascular puncture of the jugular vein, carotid and axillary arteries
- Esophageal puncture
- Pleural puncture and possible pneumothorax or intrapleural injection of local anesthetic solution
- Cervical epidural distribution of the local anesthetic, resulting in impaired ventilation and bradycardia
- Block of the laryngeal recurrent nerve, resulting in impaired arytenoid movement
- Neuropraxia
- Allergic reactions to local anesthetics
- Local anesthetic toxicity

Brachial Plexus Block: Axillary Approach

The axillary brachial plexus block aims at blocking the musculocutaneous, axillary, radial, median, and ulnar nerves in the axillary space, and has been described using either NS or US guidance.[14–17] This technique has been successfully used to provide analgesia for orthopedic surgeries involving structures located distally to the distal third of the humerus (**Figs. 3**B and **4**B), and it is associated with significant opioids and general anesthetics sparing effect.[5,18]

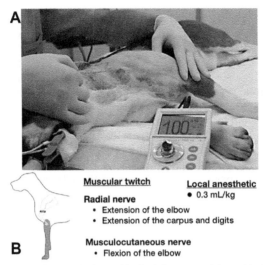

Fig. 3. NS-assisted axillary brachial plexus block. (*A*) Dog positioned in lateral recumbency with the side to be blocked uppermost. (*B*) Desensitized anatomical area. (*From* Otero, P.E. & Portela, D.A: Manual of small animal regional anesthesia: Illustrated anatomy for nerve stimulation and ultrasound-guided nerve blocks. 2nd ed. Inter-Médica S.A.I.C.I. 2019:45-134; with permission.)

Relevant anatomy

The axillary space is limited cranially by the brachiocephalicus muscle, ventrally by the pectoral muscles, laterally by the subscapularis muscle, and medially by the cervical serratus ventralis muscle.[13] Axillary vessels and nerves of the brachial plexus run in the

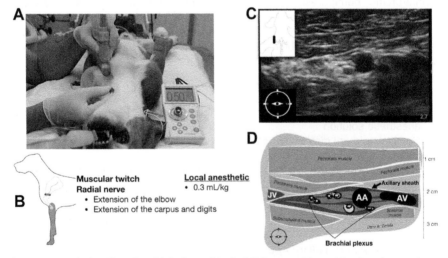

Fig. 4. US-guided axillary brachial plexus block. (*A*) Dog positioned in dorsal recumbency with the thoracic limb flexed and resting in neutral position. (*B*) Desensitized anatomical area. (*C*) US image of the brachial plexus through an axillary approach. (*D*) Schematic representation of (*C*). AA, axillary artery; AV, axillary vein; Cd, caudal; Cr, cranial; JV, jugular vein; L, lateral; M, medial. (*From* Otero, P.E. & Portela, D.A: Manual of small animal regional anesthesia: Illustrated anatomy for nerve stimulation and ultrasound-guided nerve blocks. 2nd ed. Inter-Médica S.A.I.C.I. 2019:45-134; with permission.)

axillary space, surrounded by areolar tissue and wrapped by the axillary fascia, which is the continuation of the deep fascia of the neck. Septae of the axillary fascia may separate some of the components of the brachial plexus explaining the occurrence of incomplete block when a single injection is performed.[19]

Nerve stimulation technique

A nerve stimulator can be used to assist the execution of the brachial plexus block.[14,16] Muscular responses corresponding with the stimulation of the different nerves of the plexus may be elicited when the stimulating needle enters the axillary space, and should be identified and differentiated to increase the accuracy of the blockade. An experimental study in dogs showed that the injection of 0.3 mL/kg of a local anesthetic–dye solution when the simulation of the musculocutaneous nerve was elicited, resulting in biceps brachii contraction and elbow flexion, produced sufficient distribution to achieve complete brachial plexus blockade.[16]

Technique

- Position the animal in lateral recumbency with the limb to be blocked uppermost (**Fig. 3**A).
- Introduce the needle medially to the shoulder and cranially to the acromion following a ventrocaudal direction through the brachiocephalicus muscle and parallel to the longitudinal axis of the vertebral column (see **Fig. 3**A).
- Slowly advance the needle until the target muscular contractions are elicited, ensuring the tip of the needle is cranial to the cranial border of the first rib. Two different muscular responses constitute an acceptable end point:
  - Biceps brachii contraction and elbow flexion owing to stimulation of the musculocutaneous nerve. When this response is elicited, the tip of the needle is not expected to be located in proximity to the axillary artery, decreasing the chances of accidental vascular puncture. However, an incomplete blockade of the caudal components of the brachial plexus (ulnar and medial nerves) may occur when the injection is performed in this location.
  - Triceps brachii contraction and elbow extension owing to stimulation of the radial nerve. Using this response as an end point for injection may produce a more homogeneous distribution of the local anesthetic. However, the tip of the needle may be located closer to the axillary vessels and to the thoracic inlet.
- Slowly inject 0.3 mL/kg of the selected local anesthetic when the target muscular response is elicited with a stimulating current between 0.3 to 0.5 mA.

Ultrasound-guided technique

US guidance can be used to increase the accuracy of the technique, allowing direct visualization of the target nerves and of the axillary fascia and confirmation of the correct distribution of the local anesthetic while minimizing the risks of intraneural and intravascular injection.[17]

Technique

- Position the animal in dorsal recumbency with the limb to be blocked flexed in a neutral position (**Fig. 4**A).
- The authors recommend combining this technique with NS.
- Position the linear transducer (>10 MHz) parasagittally over the axillary space, between the manubrium of the sternum and the supraglenoid tubercle of the scapula (see **Fig. 4**A).

- Sonoanatomy (**Fig. 4**C, D)
  - Adjust the transducer position until the axillary artery is identified as a pulsatile and anechoic round structure. The axillary vein is located caudally to the artery and it collapses when gentle pressure is applied to the transducer.
  - The nerves of the brachial plexus can be visualized as round structures with different degrees of echogenicity located cranially and slightly dorsally to the axillary vessels.
  - The axillary fascia can be identified as a thin hyperechoic structure surrounding the brachial plexus.
- Introduce the needle in-plane through the superficial pectoral muscle, lateral to the jugular vein and in a caudodorsal direction (see **Fig. 4**A).
- Set the nerve stimulator to 0.3 mA, 0.1 ms, and 1 Hz. When the tip of the needle is located in proximity to the target nerve, the electrical current on the NS should be increased to 0.5 mA to confirm the correct muscular response (see **Fig. 1**).
- Advance the needle through the axillary fascia until its tip reaches the dorsal aspect of the axillary artery.
- Slowly inject 0.3 mL/kg of local anesthetic solutions to ensure adequate distribution around all nerves of the plexus. During injection the tip of the needle can be gently adjusted to obtain a homogeneous spread of the local anesthetic solution around the target structures.

Potential complications

Several complications associated with axillary brachial plexus block have been reported. Nerve praxis after needle trauma or nerve compression owing to hematoma formation could result in a transient or permanent neurologic deficit. Hematomas have been reported as a complication in up to 14% of the brachial plexus blocks performed in 1 study,[20] and neurologic deficit lasting longer than 20 hours has been described after a blind brachial plexus block with 0.5% bupivacaine.[21]

Iatrogenic pneumothorax may occur if the tip of the needle is advanced past the thoracic inlet.[22] Acute onset of ventricular fibrillation was described after accidental introduction of a stimulating needle into the thoracic cavity while performing an axillary brachial plexus block.[23]

Block of the phrenic nerve and subsequent transient hemidiaphragmatic paresis is also a potential complication after axillary brachial plexus block. However, unilateral block of the phrenic nerve is usually well-tolerated in healthy animals.

Radial, Ulnar, Median and Musculocutaneous Nerves Block

The radial, ulnar, median, and musculocutaneous nerve (RUMM) block aims at blocking the musculocutaneous, radial, median, and ulnar nerves in the proximal or distal brachium region. The proximal RUMM block is performed on the proximal third of the humerus where the 4 nerves still run together, wrapped by the axillary sheath.[24] The distal RUMM block is performed in the mid-humeral region where the radial nerve is located on the lateral aspect of the brachium while the rest of the nerves run medially.[25–28] This block can be performed using the NS alone; however, the authors recommend the use of the US to increase the accuracy of the technique. The proximal approach may be used for procedures involving the distal humerus and the elbow (**Fig. 5**B), whereas the distal approach is suitable for procedures involving anatomic structures located distal to the elbow (**Fig. 6**B and **7**B).

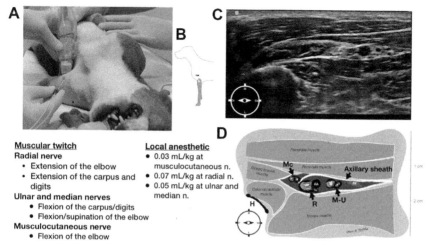

Muscular twitch
Radial nerve
• Extension of the elbow
• Extension of the carpus and digits
Ulnar and median nerves
• Flexion of the carpus/digits
• Flexion/supination of the elbow
Musculocutaneous nerve
• Flexion of the elbow

Local anesthetic
• 0.03 mL/kg at musculocutaneous n.
• 0.07 mL/kg at radial n.
• 0.05 mL/kg at ulnar and median n.

Fig. 5. US-guided proximal radial, ulnar, median and musculocutaneous (RUMM) nerve block. (A) Dog positioned in dorsal recumbency and tilted laterally to allow the target limb to rest on table. (B) Desensitized anatomical area. (C) US image of the RUMM nerves and the axillary artery through a proximal RUMM approach. (D) Schematic representation of (C). AA, axillary artery; AV, axillary vein; Cd, caudal; Cr, cranial; H, humerus; L, lateral; M, medial; Mc, musculocutaneous n.; M-U, median and ulnar n.; R, radial n. (From Otero, P.E. & Portela, D.A: Manual of small animal regional anesthesia: Illustrated anatomy for nerve stimulation and ultrasound-guided nerve blocks. 2nd ed. Inter-Médica S.A.I.C.I. 2019:45-134; with permission.)

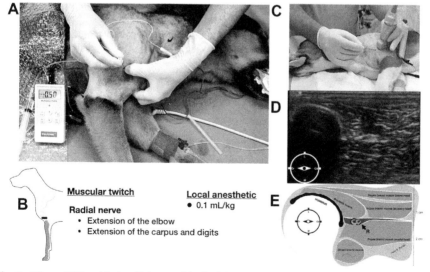

Muscular twitch
Radial nerve
• Extension of the elbow
• Extension of the carpus and digits

Local anesthetic
• 0.1 mL/kg

Fig. 6. NS- and US-guided radial nerve block. (A) Dog position for NS technique. (B) Desensitized anatomical area. (C): Dog and transducer position for US-guided technique. (D) US image of the radial nerve at the mid-humeral region. (E) Schematic representation of (D). Cd, caudal; Cr, cranial; L, lateral; M, medial; R, radial n.

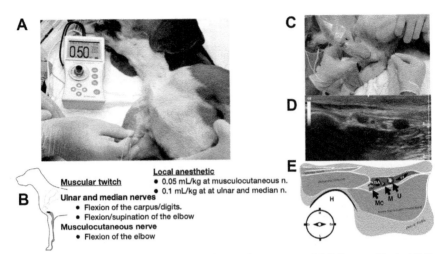

Fig. 7. NS- and US-guided ulnar median and musculocutaneous (UMM) nerve block. (*A*) Dog position for NS technique. (*B*) Desensitized anatomical area. (*C*) Dog and transducer position for US-guided technique. (*D*) US image of UMM nerves at the mid-humeral region. (*E*) Schematic representation of (*D*). Cd, caudal; Cr, cranial; L, lateral; M, medial; M, median n.; Mc, musculocutaneous n.; U, ulnar n. (*From* Otero, P.E. & Portela, D.A: Manual of small animal regional anesthesia: Illustrated anatomy for nerve stimulation and ultrasound-guided nerve blocks. 2nd ed. Inter-Médica S.A.I.C.I. 2019:45-134; with permission.)

Relevant anatomy

The RUMM nerves run on the medial aspect of the proximal humerus, caudal to the biceps brachii muscle, grouped around the axillary artery and surrounded by the axillary sheath.[13] On the middle third of the humerus the radial nerve moves laterally, and it locates among the lateral and accessory heads of the triceps brachii muscle and the brachialis muscle. On the medial aspect of the brachium, the musculocutaneous nerve runs adjacent to the caudal border of the biceps brachii muscle and cranial to the brachial artery. The median and ulnar nerves are typically located between the brachial artery and vein.

Ultrasound-guided technique

The combination of NS and US is highly recommended to increase the accuracy of nerve location while performing either of the approaches for the RUMM block.

Proximal radial, ulnar, median, and musculocutaneous nerve block

The desensitized area following a proximal RUMM block is similar to that achieved with the axillary brachial plexus block (**Fig. 5**B), and the main difference between the 2 techniques is that the former is performed on the medial surface of the humerus, which minimizes the risk of accidental vascular, pleural, and cardiac punctures, and involvement of the phrenic nerve.

Technique

- Position the animal in dorsal recumbency and slightly tilted toward the side to be blocked. The limb to be blocked should be resting on the table and the elbow should be flexed with a 90° angle (**Fig. 5**A).
- Place the linear transducer (>10 MHz) transversally on the medial aspect of the brachium, at the level of the humeral head.

- Slightly tilt the transducer to identify the biceps brachii muscle, the axillary vessels, and RUMM nerves.
- Sonoanatomy (**Fig. 5C, D**)
  - The humerus is visualized as a hyperechoic semicircle.
  - The axillary artery is identified as a hypoechoic, round, and pulsatile structure.
  - The musculocutaneous nerve is located between the biceps brachii muscle and the axillary artery.
  - The radial nerve is located lateral to the axillary artery.
  - The median–ulnar nerves are visualized as round structures located between the axillary artery and vein.
  - The axillary fascia is identified as a thin hyperechoic structure surrounding the neurovascular bundle.
  - The deep pectoral muscle can be visualized on the medial aspect of the axillary sheath.
- The insulated needle is introduced in-plane, cranial to the US transducer through the belly of the biceps brachii muscle, and directed caudally (see **Fig. 5A**).
- When the tip of the needle is in proximity to the target nerve, the electrical current on the NS should be increased to 0.5 mA to confirm the correct muscular response (see **Fig. 1**):
  - Musculocutaneous nerve: contraction of biceps brachii muscle and flexion of the elbow
  - Radial nerve: contraction of the triceps brachii muscle and extension of the elbow
  - Median–ulnar nerve trunk: contraction of the flexors of carpus and digits and flexion of carpus and digits
- A total volume 0.15 mL/kg of local anesthetic solution, divided into 3 aliquots should be injected as following:
  - Musculocutaneous nerve: 0.03 mL/kg
  - Radial nerve: 0.07 mL/kg
  - Median–ulnar trunk: 0.05 mL/kg
- The injected local anesthetic can be visualized as an anechoic structure distributing between the axillary sheath and the target nerves.

Distal radial, ulnar, median, and musculocutaneous nerve block
This block can be performed using either NS alone, or the combination of NS and US. It is performed in the midhumeral region, approaching the radial nerve on the lateral aspect of the brachium, after it leaves the common axillary sheath, and the ulnar, median, and musculocutaneous nerves on the medial aspect of the brachium.

Nerve stimulation technique
Radial nerve block
- Position the patient in lateral recumbency with the limb to be blocked uppermost and the elbow slightly flexed (**Fig. 6A**).
- The puncture site is located on the lateral aspect of the brachium, between the brachialis muscle and the lateral head of the triceps brachii muscle.
- The insulated needle is introduced perpendicularly through the lateral head of the triceps brachii muscle and caudal to the brachialis muscle until the target motor response is elicited:
  - Contraction of the triceps brachii and extension of the elbow or
  - Contraction of the extensors of the carpus and digits
- Inject 0.1 mL/kg of the local anesthetic solution.

Musculocutaneous, median, and ulnar nerves

- Position the patient in dorsal or lateral recumbency with the limb to be blocked lowermost and the elbow flexed by 90° (**Fig. 7A**).
- The puncture site is located on the medial aspect of the brachium between the biceps brachii and the medial head of the triceps brachii, and the solution is injected cranial and caudal to the brachial artery.
- Palpate the brachial artery on the distal third of the brachium between the biceps brachii and the medial head of the triceps brachii.
- Introduce the insulated needle cranially and caudally to the brachial artery to stimulate the musculocutaneous and median/ulnar nerves, respectively.
  - Musculocutaneous nerve: contraction of the brachialis and biceps brachii and flexion of the elbow
  - Median and ulnar nerves: contraction of the flexors of the carpus and digits, flexion of the carpus, and pronation of the manus
- Inject 0.05 mL/kg of local anesthetic for the musculocutaneous nerve and 0.1 mL/kg for the median and ulnar nerves.

Ultrasound-guided technique

US guidance allows identification of the target nerves and surrounding fasciae as well as confirmation of the correct local anesthetic distribution while decreasing the risk of accidental intraneural or intravascular injection. This technique can be combined with NS to confirm the correct positioning of the tip of the needle.

Ultrasound-guided radial nerve block

- Place the transducer transversally on the lateral aspect of the mid humeral region (**Fig. 6C**).
- Identify the humerus, the brachialis, and triceps brachii muscles. Adjust the transducer until the radial nerve can be visualized between these muscles (**Fig. 6D, E**).
- Introduce the needle in-plane from the cranial aspect of the brachialis muscle and direct it toward the target nerve.
- Inject 0.1 mL/kg of the local anesthetic solution.

Ultrasound-guided musculocutaneous, median, and ulnar nerves block

- Place the transducer transversally on the medial aspect of the mid humeral region (**Fig. 7C**).
- Identify the brachial artery and vein, the humerus, the brachialis and the accessory head of the triceps brachii muscle (**Fig. 7D, E**).
  - Adjust the transducer until the musculocutaneous nerve can be visualized cranially to the brachial artery and caudally to the biceps brachii muscle. The median and ulnar nerves can be visualized between the brachial artery and vein. Color flow Doppler mode may be used to differentiate the blood vessels from the nerves.
- Advance the needle in-plane, either from the cranial or from the caudal aspect of the brachium, until the target nerves are reached.
- Inject 0.05 mL/kg of local anesthetic for the musculocutaneous nerve and 0.1 mL/kg for the median and ulnar nerves.

Potential complications

- Accidental vascular puncture
- Nerve damage

Thoracic Paravertebral Blocks

Thoracic paravertebral (TPV) blocks aim at blocking the thoracic spinal nerves as they emerge from the intervertebral foramina. Local anesthetics injected into the TPV space result in nerve blockade of the dorsal and ventral rami of the respective spinal nerve, the rami communicantes, and part of the sympathetic trunk,[9] resulting in somatic and visceral analgesia of the thorax (**Fig. 11**B). Studies in humans have shown that single injections into 1 TPV space can spread longitudinally affecting several contiguous spinal nerves, and thus providing multisegmental analgesia.[29] However, studies performed in animals showed that single injections can spread longitudinally affecting several segments of the sympathetic trunk but not contiguous spinal nerves.[9,30,31] In dogs, the technique to perform TPV block has been described using either NS or US guidance.[9,31,32]

This technique is used in people to provide high-quality perioperative analgesia for thoracotomy and cranial abdominal surgeries.[33] There are no clinical studies evaluating the efficacy of this technique in veterinary patients. However, the authors of this article have been successfully using TPV blocks to provide analgesia for lateral thoracotomy or thoracic wall wounds in small animals, and anecdotally noticed a substantial reduction in the perioperative opioid requirements when this technique is used.

Relevant anatomy

The TPV spaces are located alongside the vertebral column and are limited medially by the vertebral bodies, dorsally by the internal intercostal membrane, and ventrally by the parietal pleura. The internal intercostal membrane is the continuation of the internal intercostal muscles when they approach the vertebral column. The endothoracic fascia divides the TPV space into a dorsal and a ventral compartment. The dorsal compartment contains the dorsal and ventral rami of the spinal nerves and part of the rami communicantes, while the ventral compartment contains the rami communicantes and the sympathetic trunk. The dorsal compartment communicates medially with the epidural space through the intervertebral foramen and laterally to the intercostal space. The ventral compartment of the TVP space communicates with the dorsal mediastinum and the contiguous ventral compartments of the TPV space.[9]

Nerve stimulation technique

NS can be used to assist the execution of the TPV block. When a stimulating needle is in proximity to the spinal nerve into the TPV space, the corresponding intercostal muscle twitches are elicited.[32] An experimental study performed in dogs given NS-guided injections of contrast medium showed that the injected solution remained confined in the TPV space of the injection site, suggesting that 3 to 5 contiguous spinal nerves should be blocked to obtain a wide area of desensitization.[32]

Technique

- Position the animal in sternal recumbency.
- Palpate the spinous process of the thoracic vertebra corresponding to the spinal segment to be blocked.
- Set the nerve stimulator at 1 mA (2 Hz, 0.1 ms) and introduce the stimulating needle 1 to 2 cm laterally to the spinous process through the epaxial musculature until it contacts the transverse process of the vertebra immediately caudal to the target TPV space (**Fig. 8**A).
- Withdraw the needle and walk it off on the transverse process to redirect it cranially (**Fig. 8**B, C).

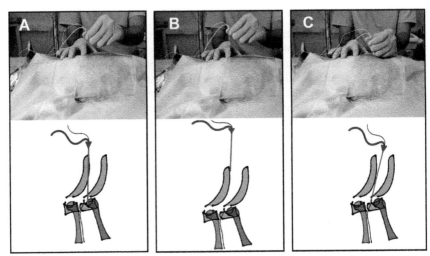

Fig. 8. Sequence for NS-assisted TPV block. (*A*) Needle introduced 1 to 2 cm laterally to the dorsal midline until it contacts the transverse process of the vertebra caudal to the target level. (*B*) The needle was withdrawn to adjust its angle. (*C*) The needle was reintroduced and redirected to be walked off cranially on the transverse process and advanced until the intercostal muscular twitch is elicited. (*From* Otero, P.E. & Portela, D.A: Manual of small animal regional anesthesia: Illustrated anatomy for nerve stimulation and ultrasound-guided nerve blocks. 2nd ed. Inter-Médica S.A.I.C.I. 2019:219-272; with permission.)

- Advance the needle slowly into the TPV space until the tip of the needle is in proximity to the spinal nerve, as suggested by the contraction of the intercostal or the abdominal muscles.
- Gradually decrease the current intensity until the muscular twitch can be elicited with an electrical current > 0.3 and ≤ 0.5 mA.
- Aspirate to rule out the presence of blood or air and inject 0.05 to 0.1 mL/kg of the local anesthetic solution.
- Repeat the procedure on 1 or 2 cranial and caudal spinal levels.

Ultrasound-guided technique

US guidance can be used to increase the accuracy of TPV injections, allowing direct visualization of the TPV space, the needle, and the correct distribution of the injected solution.[9]

Technique

- Position the animal in sternal recumbency (**Fig. 9**A).
- Identify the spinal segments to be blocked by counting the intercostal spaces using the US, and following the corresponding rib dorsally until the transducer is positioned parasagittally 1 to 2 cm to the dorsal midline, with a slight oblique orientation (see **Fig. 9**A).
- High-frequency (>10 MHz) linear transducers are recommended. For large dogs where the TPV space is deeper that 6 cm, convex transducers may be needed.
- The authors recommend using 20G, 90-mm Tuohy needle attached to an extension line or a T-port. The Tuohy needle helps perceiving the perforation of the internal intercostal membrane and may decrease the risk of accidently piercing the parietal pleura.

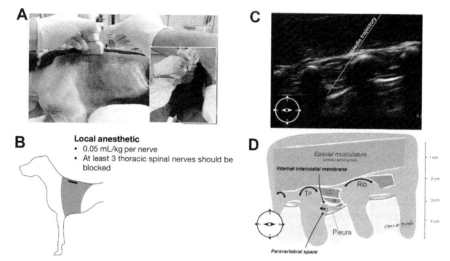

Fig. 9. US-guided TPV block. (*A*) Dog and transducer position. (*B*) desensitized anatomical area. (*C*) US image of the TPV space and needle trajectory. (*D*) Schematic representation of (*C*). Cd, caudal; Cr, cranial; EI, external intercostal muscle; II, internal intercostal muscle; L, lateral; LC, levatores costarum muscle; M, medial; TP, transverse process. (*From* Otero, P.E. & Portela, D.A: Manual of small animal regional anesthesia: Illustrated anatomy for nerve stimulation and ultrasound-guided nerve blocks. 2nd ed. Inter-Médica S.A.I.C.I. 2019:219-272; with permission.)

- Sonoanatomy of the TPV space (**Fig. 9**C, D)
  - Two consecutive transverse processes are identified as hyperechoic structures with an acoustic shadow underneath. When the transducer is positioned with a slight oblique orientation, a transverse process will be visualized cranially and a rib caudally
  - The parietal pleura can be identified as a hyperechoic line between the 2 acoustic shadows of the transverse processes. The sliding sign of the visceral pleura can also be identified during respiratory movements.
  - The internal intercostal membrane can be identified as a thin hyperechoic line, located between the parietal pleura and the external intercostal muscle, connecting 2 transverse processes.
  - The TPV space has a triangular shape and is located between 2 consecutive transverse processes, ventral to the internal intercostal membrane and dorsal to the parietal pleura (see **Fig. 9**D).
- Introduce the needle in-plane from the caudal margin of the transducer (**Fig. 9**A–C). The needle is advanced through the epaxial muscle, the levatores costarum, the external intercostal muscle, and finally the internal intercostal membrane.
- Position the tip of the needle between the internal intercostal membrane and the parietal pleura (ie, within the TPV space).
- Inject 0.05 to 0.1 mL/kg of local anesthetic. Ventral displacement of the pleura during injection indicates that the local anesthetic is administered at target.
- Repeat the procedure on 1 cranial and caudal spinal levels.

Potential complications
Epidural spread of local anesthetic solution has been reported as a complication in experimental studies.[30,32] Accidental parietal pleura puncture may lead to intrapleural injection of local anesthetic or pneumothorax.

Intercostal Nerve Blocks

Intercostal nerves blocks can be used to provide desensitization of the thoracic wall. As opposed to the TPV block, this approach does not involve the dorsal branches of the spinal nerves or the rami communicantes. Therefore, intercostal nerve blocks are not expected to provide any visceral analgesia and the desensitized area is limited to the ventrolateral aspect of the thoracic wall (**Fig. 10**B).

Intercostal nerve blocks have been reported to provide comparable analgesia to epidural and systemic opioid administration in dogs undergoing lateral thoracotomy.[34,35] This nerve block also resulted in improved ventilatory function compared with the systemic administration of opioids in canine patients undergoing thoracotomy.[36] No studies have been performed to compare the analgesic effect of intercostal nerve blocks with regional anesthesia strategies expected to offer a wider area of desensitization and visceral analgesia (ie, thoracic epidural injections and TPV blocks) in animals undergoing lateral thoracotomy.

Intercostal nerve blocks are technically simple to perform and can be used to provide analgesia in a variety of clinical scenarios including thoracostomy tube placement, medial sternotomy (bilateral intercostal nerve blocks T2–T9), mastectomy of the thoracic mammary glands, thoracic wall wounds or mass removals, and pain management for rib fractures.

Relevant anatomy

The intercostal nerves run along the caudal aspect of each rib, in proximity to the intercostal artery and vein, deep to the intercostal muscles and separated from the parietal pleura by the endothoracic fascia. Their cutaneous and ventral branches innervate the ventrolateral aspect of the thoracic wall (see **Fig. 10**B).

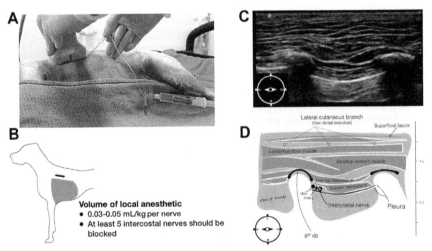

Volume of local anesthetic
- 0.03-0.05 mL/kg per nerve
- At least 5 intercostal nerves should be blocked

Fig. 10. US-guided intercostal nerve block. (*A*) Dog and transducer position. (*B*) desensitized anatomical area. (*C*) US image of the intercostal space. (*D*) Schematic representation of (*C*). Cd, caudal; Cr, cranial; L, lateral; M, medial. (*From* Otero, P.E. & Portela, D.A: Manual of small animal regional anesthesia: Illustrated anatomy for nerve stimulation and ultrasound-guided nerve blocks. 2nd ed. Inter-Médica S.A.I.C.I. 2019:219-272; with permission.)

Ultrasound-guided technique

Although this block is commonly performed blindly, positioning the needle tip on the caudomedial aspect of the rib, US guidance can be used to confirm the injection is being performed at target and to decrease the likelihood of accidental pleural puncture.

Technique

- Position the animal in lateral, sternal, or dorsal recumbency.
- The authors recommend using 22G, 50- to 75-mm Quincke spinal or Tuohy needle. The use of a blunt Tuohy needle reduces the risks of accidently advancing the needle through the parietal pleura.
- Place the linear US transducer (>10 MHz) transversally to the ribs (**Fig. 10**A).
- Sonoanatomy of the intercostal space (**Fig. 10**C, D)
  ○ The ribs are identified as semiround hyperechoic structures projecting an acoustic shadow.
  ○ The parietal pleura is recognized as a hyperechoic line connecting 2 consecutive ribs.
  ○ The intercostal nerves cannot be directly visualized, but they lie on the caudal aspect of each rib, superficially to the parietal pleura and deep to the internal intercostal muscle.
- Introduce the needle in-plane from the caudal aspect of the transducer and direct it toward the caudal aspect of the target rib until the tip is positioned between the internal intercostal muscle and the parietal pleura (see **Fig. 10**A). Performing the block on the proximal third of the rib ensures the lateral cutaneous branch of the spinal nerve is involved.
- Displacement of the parietal pleura away from the needle tip while performing the injection confirms correct injection site.
- Inject a volume of 0.03 to 0.05 mL/kg per point.

Potential complications

Although specific veterinary studies evaluating the complications with this technique are lacking, potential complications include pneumothorax, accidental intravascular or intrapleural injection, nerve injury, and local anesthetic toxicity when several intercostal nerves are blocked.

Erector Spinae Plane Block

The erector spinae plane block is a technique recently described in humans to treat acute and chronic thoracic and lumbar pain.[37,38] This block aims at desensitizing the medial and lateral branches of the dorsal rami of the spinal nerves. The proposed mechanism of action for this block involves the multisegmental spread of the injectate in a fascial plane formed by the erector spinae muscles and transverse processes and lamina of the vertebrae.[37,39]

Although veterinary research studies on this novel technique are still underway, potential applications for this block may include its use in dogs undergoing hemilaminectomy or any painful procedure involving the dorsum.[40] This technique may be performed bilaterally. However, unilateral injections should be sufficient to block the surgical area in animals undergoing hemilaminectomy.

Relevant anatomy

The dorsal rami leave the spinal nerves and travel dorsally between the erector spinae muscles and the transvers process of the vertebrae. The erector spinae muscle group comprises the iliocostalis, longissimus, spinalis, and semispinalis thoracis muscles.[41] The dorsal rami divide into a medial and a lateral branch. The medial branch travels between the longissimus thoracis and the multifidus muscles and innervates the epaxial muscles, the vertebral lamina and the facet joints[42]; the lateral branch travels laterally between the longissimus thoracis and the iliocostalis thoracis, innervating the epaxial muscles and the skin of the dorsolateral aspect of the thoracic wall (**Fig 11**B).

Ultrasound-guided technique
This technique should be performed under US guidance to ensure correct needle positioning and to visualize the distribution of the injected solution in the correct fascial plane.

Technique
- Position the animal in sternal recumbency.
- Position the transducer (>10 MHz) longitudinally over the epiaxial musculature with a parasagittal orientation (**Fig. 11**A).
- Identify the target vertebral segment. The authors recommend performing the injection one vertebral space cranial to the target segment.
- Sonoanatomy of the erector spinae plane (**Fig. 11**C, D)
  - The thoracic transverse processes are identified as hyperechoic structures ventral to the epaxial muscles, projecting an acoustic shadow.
  - The transducer should be slid laterally and medially to detect the lateral edge of the transverse process (see **Fig. 11**D).
  - The parietal pleura can be visualized as a hyperechoic line deep and in between 2 consecutives transverse processes. This landmark should always be identified to decrease the risk of accidental intrathoracic puncture.
- The authors recommend using a 20G, 90-mm Tuohy needle attached to a prefilled extension line or a T-port. The needle should be introduced in-plane through the epaxial muscles and advanced until its tip contacts the lateral portion of the dorsal aspect of the target transverse process (see **Fig. 11**C).

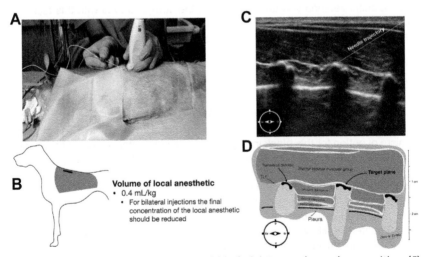

Fig. 11. US-guided erector spinae plane (ESP) block. (*A*) Dog and transducer position. (*B*) desensitized anatomical area. (*C*) US image of the ESP and needle trajectory. (*D*) Schematic representation of (*C*). Cd, caudal; Cr, cranial; L, lateral; M, medial; TLF, thoracolumbar fascia. (*From* Otero, P.E. & Portela, D.A: Manual of small animal regional anesthesia: Illustrated anatomy for nerve stimulation and ultrasound-guided nerve blocks. 2nd ed. Inter-Médica S.A.I.C.I. 2019:219-272; with permission.)

- Inject 0.4 mL/kg of the local anesthetic solution, which should be observed spreading cranial and caudal between the transverse process and the erector spinae muscular group. For unilateral injections, bupivacaine or ropivacaine 0.5% are recommended. For bilateral injections, the final concentration of the local anesthetic should be reduced to avoid exceeding the maximum recommended dose for each species

Potential complications

There are no studies evaluating the potential complications of this technique in animals. Epidural spread and pneumothorax are reported complication in humans after this block.

SUMMARY

The field of small animal regional anesthesia has expanded significantly, and multiple techniques to desensitize the thoracic limb and thorax have been described recently. These techniques are implemented routinely in clinical practice and offer a valuable contribution to multimodal anesthesia strategies, allowing a significant decrease in perioperative systemic analgesic consumption. Although no large-scale studies evaluating the complications associated with regional anesthesia in small animals are available, based on the current literature and on the authors' clinical experience, these techniques are effective and safe when performed correctly. The use of objective methods of nerve location and adequate equipment, including needles designed specifically for regional anesthesia, is strongly encouraged to reduce the subjectivity and increase the accuracy of blind techniques, and to decrease the risks of complications, respectively.

REFERENCES

1. Munirama S, McLeod G. A systematic review and meta-analysis of ultrasound versus electrical stimulation for peripheral nerve location and blockade. Anaesthesia 2015;70(9):1084–91.
2. Marhofer P, Fritsch G. Safe performance of peripheral regional anaesthesia: the significance of ultrasound guidance. Anaesthesia 2017;72(4):431–4.
3. Portela DA, Verdier N, Otero PE. Regional anesthetic techniques for the thoracic limb and thorax in small animals: a review of the literature and technique description. Vet J 2018;241:8–19.
4. Portela DA, Verdier N, Otero PE. Regional anesthetic techniques for the pelvic limb and abdominal wall in small animals: a review of the literature and technique description. Vet J 2018;238:27–40.
5. Mosing M, Reich H, Moens Y. Clinical evaluation of the anaesthetic sparing effect of brachial plexus block in cats. Vet Anaesth Analg 2010;37(2):154–61.
6. Romano M, Portela DA, Breghi G, et al. Stress-related biomarkers in dogs administered regional anaesthesia or fentanyl for analgesia during stifle surgery. Vet Anaesth Analg 2016;43(1):44–54.
7. Thiyagarajan S, Velraj J, Hussain Ahmed MI, et al. Subarachnoid block with continuous TAP catheter analgesia produces less chronic pain and better functional outcome after inguinal hernioplasty: a randomized controlled observer-blinded study. Reg Anesth Pain Med 2019;44(2):228–33.
8. Schroeder CA, Snyder LBC, Tearney CC, et al. Ultrasound-guided transversus abdominis plane block in the dog: an anatomical evaluation. Vet Anaesth Analg 2011;38(3):267–71.

9. Portela DA, Campoy L, Otero PE, et al. Ultrasound-guided thoracic paravertebral injection in dogs: a cadaveric study. Vet Anaesth Analg 2017;44(3):636–45.

10. Hadzic A, Dilberovic F, Shah S, et al. Combination of intraneural injection and high injection pressure leads to fascicular injury and neurologic deficits in dogs. Reg Anesth Pain Med 2004;29(5):417–23.

11. Otero PE, Fuensalida SE, Briganti A, et al. Ultrasound-guided subscalenic brachial plexus block in dogs: a cadaveric study. Proceeding of the spring meeting of the Association of Veterinary Anaesthetists Manchester, UK. Vet Anaesth Analg 2017;44:983–8.

12. Fuensalida S, Ceballos M, Verdier N, et al. Sonographic evaluation of diaphragm function during a subscalenic brachial plexus block in dogs: technique and clinical applications. Proceeding of the spring meeting of the Association of Veterinary Anaesthetists Manchester, UK. Vet Anaesth Analg 2017;44:983–8.

13. Evans HE, de Lahunta A. Chapter 17 - The spinal nerves. In: Evans HE, de Lahunta A, editors. Miller's anatomy of the dog. 4th edition. St Louis (MI): Elsevier Saunders; 2013. p. 611–57.

14. Mahler SP, Adogwa AO. Anatomical and experimental studies of brachial plexus, sciatic, and femoral nerve-location using peripheral nerve stimulation in the dog. Vet Anaesth Analg 2008;35(1):80–9.

15. Futema F, Fantoni D, Auler J Jr, et al. A new brachial plexus block technique in dogs. Vet Anaesth Analg 2002;29(3):133–9.

16. Campoy L, Martin-Flores M, Looney AL, et al. Distribution of a lidocaine-methylene blue solution staining in brachial plexus, lumbar plexus and sciatic nerve blocks in the dog. Vet Anaesth Analg 2008;35(4):348–54.

17. Campoy L, Bezuidenhout AJ, Gleed RD, et al. Ultrasound-guided approach for axillary brachial plexus, femoral nerve, and sciatic nerve blocks in dogs. Vet Anaesth Analg 2010;37(2):144–53.

18. Ansón A, Laredo FG, Gil F, et al. Evaluation of an ultrasound-guided technique for axillary brachial plexus blockade in cats. J Feline Med Surg 2017;19(2):146–52.

19. Moens NM, Caulkett NA. The use of a catheter to provide brachial plexus block in dogs. Can Vet J 2000;41(9):685–9.

20. Ricco C, Shih A, Killos M, et al. Different volumes of injectate using electrostimulator and blinded techniques for brachial plexus block in dogs. Vet Rec 2013; 173(24):608.

21. Ridge P. Complication following a brachial plexus block. Vet Rec 2014; 174(24):614.

22. Bhalla RJ, Leece EA. Pneumothorax following nerve stimulator-guided axillary brachial plexus block in a dog. Vet Anaesth Analg 2015;42(6):658–9.

23. Adami C, Studer N. A case of severe ventricular arrhythmias occurring as a complication of nerve-stimulator guided brachial plexus location. Vet Anaesth Analg 2015;42(2):230–1.

24. Tayari H, Otero P, Rossetti A, et al. Proximal RUMM block in dogs: preliminary results of cadaveric and clinical study. Vet Anaesth Analg 2019. https://doi.org/10.1016/j.vaa.2018.11.009.

25. Trumpatori BJ, Carter JE, Hash J, et al. Evaluation of a midhumeral block of the radial, ulnar, musculocutaneous and median (RUMM block) nerves for analgesia of the distal aspect of the thoracic limb in dogs. Vet Surg 2010;39(7):785–96.

26. Bortolami E, Love EJ, Harcourt-Brown TR, et al. Use of mid-humeral block of the radial, ulnar, musculocutaneous and median (RUMM block) nerves for extensor carpi radialis muscle biopsy in a conscious dog with generalized neuromuscular disease. Vet Anaesth Analg 2012;39(4):446–7.

27. Portela DA, Raschi A, Otero PE. Ultrasound guided mid-humeral block of the radial, ulnar, median and musculocutaneous (RUMM block) nerves in a dog with traumatic exposed metacarpal luxation. Vet Anaesth Analg 2013;40(5): 552–4.

28. Castiñeiras D, Viscasillas J, Seymour C. A modified approach for performing ultrasound-guided radial, ulnar, median and musculocutaneous nerve block in a dog. Vet Anaesth Analg 2015;42(6):659–61.

29. Saito T, Den S, Cheema SP, et al. A single-injection, multi-segmental paravertebral block-extension of somatosensory and sympathetic block in volunteers. Acta Anaesthesiol Scand 2001;45(1):30–3.

30. Monticelli P, Jones I, Viscasillas J. Ultrasound-guided thoracic paravertebral block: cadaveric study in foxes (Vulpes vulpes). Vet Anaesth Analg 2017;44(4): 968–72.

31. Ferreira TH, Teixeira LBC, Schroeder CA, et al. Description of an ultrasound-guided thoracic paravertebral block technique and the spread of dye in dog cadavers. Vet Anaesth Analg 2018;45(6):811–9.

32. Portela DA, Otero PE, Sclocco M, et al. Anatomical and radiological study of the thoracic paravertebral space in dogs: iohexol distribution pattern and use of the nerve stimulator. Vet Anaesth Analg 2012;39(4):398–408.

33. Richardson J, Lonnqvist P. Thoracic paravertebral block. Br J Anaesth 1998;81: 230–8.

34. Flecknell PA, Kirk AJ, Liles JH, et al. Post-operative analgesia following thoracotomy in the dog: an evaluation of the effects of bupivacaine intercostal nerve block and nalbuphine on respiratory function. Lab Anim 1991;25(4):319–24.

35. Pascoe PJ, Dyson DH. Analgesia after lateral thoracotomy in dogs. Epidural morphine vs. intercostal bupivacaine. Vet Surg 1993;22(2):141–7.

36. Thompson SE, Johnson JM. Analgesia in dogs after intercostal thoracotomy. A comparison of morphine, selective intercostal nerve block, and interpleural regional analgesia with bupivacaine. Vet Surg 1991;20(1):73–7.

37. Forero M, Adhikary SD, Lopez H, et al. The erector spinae plane block: a novel analgesic technique in thoracic neuropathic pain. Reg Anesth Pain Med 2016; 41(5):621–7.

38. Tsui BCH, Fonseca A, Munshey F, et al. The erector spinae plane (ESP) block: a pooled review of 242 cases. J Clin Anesth 2018;53:29–34.

39. Schoenfeldt J, Guffey R, Fingerman M. Cadaveric study investigating the mechanism of action of erector spinae blockade. Reg Anesth Pain Med 2019. https://doi.org/10.1136/rapm-2018-100190.

40. Portela DA, Fuensalida S, Viscasillas J, et al. Section 4: peripheral nerve blocks of the thorax and abdomen. In: Otero PE, Portela DA, editors. Manual of small animal regional anesthesia: illustrated anatomy for nerve stimulation and ultrasound-guided nerve blocks. 2nd edition. Ciudad Autonoma de Buenos Aires (Argentina): Editorial Inter-Médica; 2019. p. 219–72.

41. Hermanson JW. Chapter 6 - The muscular system. In: Evans HE, de Lahunta A, editors. Miller's anatomy of the dog. 4th edition. St Louis (MI): Elsevier Saunders; 2013. p. 185–280.

42. Forsythe WB, Ghoshal NG. Innervation of the canine thoracolumbar vertebral column. Anat Rec 1984;208(1):57–63.

Locoregional Anesthesia for Hind Limbs

Luis Campoy, LV CertVA, MRCVS

KEYWORDS

- Local anesthetic • Ultrasound guidance • Peripheral nerve block • Pelvic limb

KEY POINTS

- The provision of good-quality analgesia during surgical procedures involving the pelvic limb without the use of opioids is possible with the use of regional anesthetic techniques.
- Sound anatomic knowledge is needed to master these techniques.
- The use of ultrasound guidance seems to be superior to any other technique and even with identified and known deficiencies, is now considered the gold standard.

OVERVIEW

The field of locoregional anesthesia is being reinvigorated by the traction that opioid-free anesthesia and analgesia is gaining. Three recently published reviews regarding veterinary locoregional anesthesia provide good evidence of the current situation.[1–3] Locoregional techniques are showing promising results to improve analgesia, reduce opioid requirements,[4] and improve early postoperative recovery.[5]

Ultrasound guidance is believed to be superior to any other technique, including electrolocation,[6] and is currently considered the gold standard when performing peripheral nerve blocks.[7] Ultrasound guidance is still not perfect; equipment-related and operator-related shortcomings still exist.[8] Equipment limitations include correct visualization of deep structures and narrow ultrasound windows; operator factors include proximity to the nerve or the operator's perception and interpretation of needle-to-nerve proximity and the search for the "sweet spot" (how close is too close) to deliver the local anesthetic. In this article, only ultrasound-guided techniques are described.

In the last decade, several articles describing various approaches and clinical use of the lumbar and sacral plexus block (preiliac and parasacral approaches),[9–19] saphenous nerve block,[19,20] and sciatic nerve block[21] using ultrasound guidance have

Disclosure Statement: The author has no relationship with a commercial company that has a direct financial interest in the subject matter or materials discussed in this article or with a company making a competing product.
Department of Clinical Sciences, Cornell University, College of Veterinary Medicine, Mailbox 32, Ithaca, NY 14853, USA
E-mail address: luis.campoy@cornell.edu

been published. It is clear that in-depth anatomic knowledge of the relevant sites is important to not only perform but also understand the nuances of these techniques.

The lumbosacral plexus serves the entire pelvic limb, and it is formed by the ventral branches of L3 to S3. The nerves that form this plexus include (from cranial to caudal) the ilioinguinal, genitofemoral, lateral cutaneous femoral, iliopsoas, femoral, obturator, cranial gluteal, caudal gluteal, sciatic, gemelli, internal obturator, caudal cutaneous femoral, pelvic, superficial perineal, pudendal, levator ani, coccygeous, branch to caudal nerve trunk.[22]

A combined femoral (preiliac approach) and sciatic (parasacral/transgluteal) nerve block is appropriate for a variety of procedures, including pelvic limb amputations, hemipelvic fracture repairs, and articular procedures (femoral head osteotomies). A combined saphenous and sciatic (caudal approach) allows surgery on the stifle, such as arthroscopies, anterior cruciate ligament repair, tibial plateau leveling osteotomy (TPLO), tibial tuberosity advancement (TTA), or surgery involving the tibia, such as a fracture repair. Finally, a sciatic nerve block alone is sufficient to perform surgery of the foot and the ankle (hock), such as hock arthrodesis or even laceration repairs of the ischiotibial muscles (as long as the caudal gluteal branch is blocked as is the case with a transgluteal approach).

PREILIAC/SUPRAINGUINAL APPROACH

A preiliac/suprainguinal approach to the femoral nerve aims to deliver the local anesthetic solution within the belly of the iliopsoas muscle in proximity to the intramuscular course of the femoral nerve.[9,10,15,16] This approach blocks the hemipelvis (when combined with a transgluteal approach to the sciatic nerve) and the entire femur. It therefore provides adequate analgesia for surgical procedures such as pelvic limb amputation, femoral head osteotomies, and femoral fracture repairs.

Relevant Anatomy

The femoral nerve originates at the ventral spinal branches of L4, L5, and L6 (**Fig. 1**). The spinal nerves anastomose and join to form the femoral nerve. The femoral nerve runs in a caudal direction within the iliopsoas muscle. At this location, the femoral nerve is in close relation with the external iliac artery.

Ultrasound Anatomy

With the dog in dorsal recumbency, the ultrasound transducer should be positioned over the lateral abdomen at the level of L5 to L7 to obtain a short axis view of the

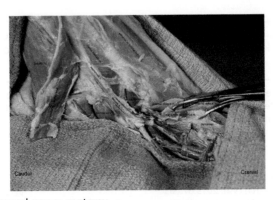

Fig. 1. Preiliac femoral nerve: anatomy.

iliopsoas muscle (**Fig. 2**). The pulse of the external iliac artery can be easily identified. The femoral nerve is located within the belly of the iliopsoas muscle. As the transducer is glided from cranial to caudal, the femoral nerve can be seen in its short axis, shifting its position from the far field to the near field as the transducer is moved caudally corresponding to the femoral nerve emerging from the intervertebral foramina, entering the iliopsoas muscle, and finally leaving the iliopsoas muscle through the muscular lacuna.

Procedure

With the dog in dorsal recumbency the ventrolateral aspect of the abdomen should be clipped and surgically prepared (**Fig. 3**). The puncture site should be in a preiliac location in-plane with the transducer. A 100 mm 20G insulated needle should be advanced toward the femoral nerve. If using combined electrolocation, a quadriceps muscle twitch should be observed at 0.3 mA once the tip of the needle is in close proximity to the femoral nerve. A volume of 0.2 to 0.4 mL kg^{-1} of local anesthetic solution has been recommended.

SAPHENOUS NERVE BLOCK

This block, when used in combination with a sciatic nerve block, can provide analgesia for procedures involving the stifle, such as knee arthroscopies, TPLO, TTA, extracapsular repairs, meniscectomies, patellar tendon ruptures, or luxating patella among others. In addition, it can provide analgesia in severe cases of osteoarthritis of the stifle.

Relevant Anatomy

The saphenous nerve is a sensory branch of the femoral nerve (**Fig. 4**). It arises from the femoral nerve as soon as the femoral nerve leaves the iliopsoas muscle through the muscular lacuna. Subsequently, it courses along deep to the caudal belly of the sartorius muscle. At the level of the midthigh, it courses distally superficial to the

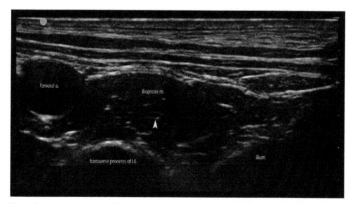

Fig. 2. Preiliac femoral nerve: ultrasound. An ultrasound image obtained by placing the ultrasound transducer over the lateral abdomen perpendicular to the direction of the spine and at the level of L6, just cranial to the ilium. Note that the ultrasound marker is located cranially. A short axis view of the iliopsoas muscle at the level of L6 can be observed. The external iliac artery can be identified medially. The femoral nerve is located within the belly of the iliopsoas muscle (*arrowhead*). The acoustic shadows cast by the ilium (lateral) and the transverse process of L6 (medial) can be observed.

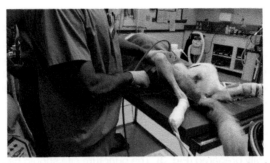

Fig. 3. Preiliac femoral nerve block: procedure. Preiliac approach to the femoral nerve with the patient positioned in dorsal recumbency. Also note the position of the ultrasound transducer with the marker oriented medially. The needle is in-plane with the transducer.

vastus medialis muscle, embedded within a sheath of fibrous tissue together with the vein and femoral artery.

Ultrasound Anatomy

The ultrasound transducer should be positioned in the medial aspect of the midthigh to obtain a short axis view of the femoral artery (**Fig. 5**). The femoral artery should be observed deep to the sartorius muscle, between the vastus medialis and the adductor muscles. The saphenous nerve is located within the neurovascular bundle, seen as a nodular hypoechoic structure caudal to the femoral artery.

Procedure

The patient should be positioned in lateral recumbency, with the pelvic limb to be blocked positioned uppermost, abducted 90°, and extended caudally (**Fig. 6**). The leg to be blocked should be clipped and surgically prepared. The ultrasound transducer should be oriented perpendicular to the course of the femoral artery so that a short axis view of the neurovascular bundle can be observed. The needle should be advanced in-plane with the transducer through the vastus medialis muscle aiming

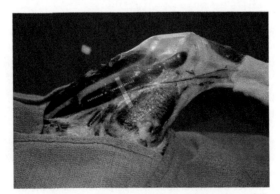

Fig. 4. Saphenous nerve: anatomy. Dissection of the medial aspect of the thigh of a dog in lateral recumbency with the left leg adducted 90° and extended caudally. Note the rectangular overlay shape representing the ultrasound transducer footprint. The caudal part of the sartorius muscle is covering the femoral artery and vein and the saphenous nerve. The neurovascular bundle runs along the medial surface of the. vastus medialis muscle.

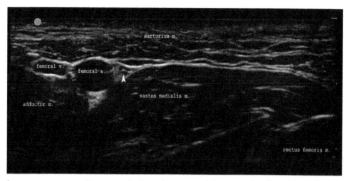

Fig. 5. Saphenous nerve: ultrasound. An ultrasound image obtained by placing the ultrasound transducer perpendicular to the course of the femoral artery at the level of the medial aspect of the midthigh. Note the marker in a caudal position. A short axis view of the neurovascular bundle can be observed. Note the arrowhead indicating the location of the saphenous nerve inside the neurovascular bundle. Note the vastus medialis muscle deep and cranial and the adductor muscle deep and caudal to the neurovascular bundle. The caudal part of the sartorius muscle lies right on top.

toward the cranial aspect of the femoral artery until the tip is located within the neurovascular sheath. An aliquot of the local anesthetic solution may be administered to observe the compression of the arterial wall, indicating correct positioning of the needle. A volume of 0.1 mL kg^{-1} is most commonly used by the author. It is important to realize that this block does not cause paralysis of the quadriceps group.

LUMBOSACRAL TRUNK/SCIATIC NERVE (PARASACRAL/TRANSGLUTEAL APPROACH)

This technique blocks the sciatic nerve at its origin at a location proximal to the cranial gluteal nerve and therefore produces anesthesia of the gluteal and ischiotrochanteric muscles (internal obturator, gemelli, quadratus femoris muscles) and the gluteal muscles as well as the ischiotibial muscles (biceps femoris, semimembranosus, semitendinosus); when combined with a lumbar plexus block, almost the entire hip can be blocked (the sensitive innervation of the canine hip joint involves the cranial gluteal nerve, obturator nerve, the sciatic nerve, and the femoral nerve[23,24]).

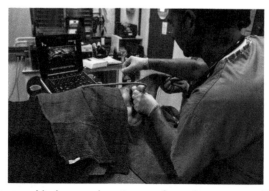

Fig. 6. Saphenous nerve block: procedure. Image of a saphenous nerve block being carried out. Note that the patient is positioned in lateral recumbency with the leg to be blocked adducted 90° and extended caudally.

Relevant Anatomy

The sciatic nerve is formed by the ventral branches of the L6, L7, and S1 spinal nerves (**Fig. 7**). The lumbosacral trunk is located medial to the ilium, deep to the midgluteal muscle and in close relation to the gluteal vessels.

Ultrasound Anatomy

With the transducer positioned between the sacral crest and the iliac wing, a short axis view of the lumbosacral trunk should be obtained (**Fig. 8**). The lumbosacral trunk can be observed deep to the superficial and midgluteal muscle, between the wing of the ilium and the sacral crest.

Procedure

With the dog in lateral recumbency and with the site to be blocked uppermost, the ultrasound transducer should be positioned over the gluteal muscles to obtain a short axis view of the lumbosacral trunk (**Fig. 9**). The needle should be advanced in-plane with the ultrasound transducer and directed from medial to lateral. If electrolocation is being used, a biceps femoris, hamstring, foot flexor, and extensor muscles or a combination thereof may be elicited. A volume of 0.1 to 0.2 mL kg^{-1} of local anesthetic has been suggested.

SCIATIC (CAUDAL APPROACH)

This approach is commonly used in combination with a saphenous nerve block for procedures involving the stifle. It can be used as a stand-alone block for procedures involving the hock or the foot (except the first toe).

Relevant Anatomy

The sciatic nerve descends the pelvic limb between the greater trochanter and the ischiatic tuberosity (**Fig. 10**). Distal to the greater trochanter and ischiatic tuberosity, the sciatic nerve lies caudal to the femur in a channel formed by the biceps femoris muscle laterally, the semimembranosus muscle caudomedially, and the adductor muscle medially.

Ultrasound Anatomy

The ultrasound transducer should be positioned over the lateral aspect of the thigh, distal to the ischiatic tuberosity and oriented in a craniocaudal position; a short axis

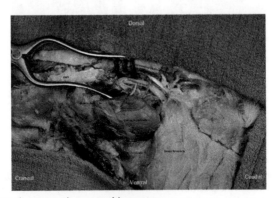

Fig. 7. Sciatic nerve (parasacral approach): anatomy.

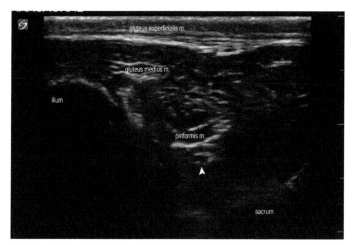

Fig. 8. Sciatic nerve (parasacral approach): ultrasound. Note the arrowhead pointing at the lumbosacral trunk

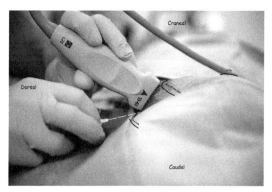

Fig. 9. Sciatic nerve (parasacral approach): procedure.

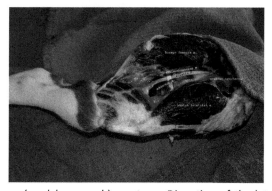

Fig. 10. Sciatic nerve (caudal approach): anatomy. Dissection of the lateral aspect of the right pelvic limb. The biceps femoris muscle has been disinserted from its cranial attachment to the vastus lateralis muscle and has been reflected caudally to expose the sciatic nerve. Note the rectangular overlay shape representing the ultrasound transducer footprint.

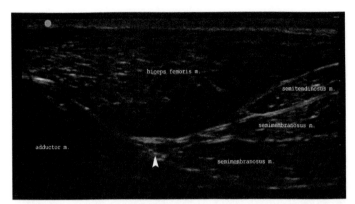

Fig. 11. Sciatic nerve (caudal approach): ultrasound. An ultrasound image obtained by placing the ultrasound transducer perpendicular and caudal to the femur in the lateral aspect of the midthigh. Note the marker is located in a cranial position. The arrowhead indicates the sciatic nerve. The nerve can be seen as a double-discoid hypoechoic shape.

view of the sciatic nerve should be obtained (**Fig. 11**). The biceps femoris muscle can be observed superficial (lateral) to the sciatic nerve (near field). The semitendinosus muscle can be seen in a caudal location. Deep (medial) to the biceps femoris is the adductor muscle. The semimembranosus muscle is located caudal and deep (medial) to the biceps femoris. The sciatic nerve can be seen as a small discoid or double-discoid hyperechoic structure, located deep (medial) to the biceps femoris muscle.

Procedure

With the patient in lateral recumbency with the leg to be blocked positioned upper-most and extended naturally, the ultrasound transducer should be positioned over the lateral aspect of the thigh distal to the greater trochanter and ischiatic tuberosity to obtain a short axis view of the sciatic nerve (**Fig. 12**). The needle puncture site is located in the caudal aspect in-plane with the ultrasound transducer. The needle

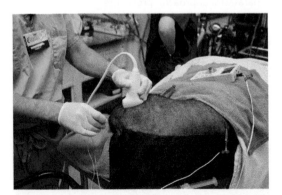

Fig. 12. Sciatic nerve (caudal approach): procedure. Image of a sciatic nerve block being carried out. Note that the patient is positioned in lateral recumbency with the leg to be blocked extended in a natural position. Note the positioning of the ultrasound transducer over the biceps femoris muscle perpendicular to the course of the sciatic nerve. Note the needle in a caudal position over the semimembranosus muscle, in-plane with the ultrasound transducer.

should be advanced in-plane with the ultrasound transducer toward the sciatic nerve, keeping the needle tip in the ultrasound field of view at all times. If electrolocation is used in combination with ultrasound guidance, either dorsiflexion or plantar extension (most commonly seen) of the foot should be observed when the tip of the needle is located in the proximity of the peroneal (dorsiflexion) or tibial (plantar extension) branches. Local anesthetic solution can be injected. A volume of 0.1 mL kg^{-1} is most commonly used by the author.

REFERENCES

1. Portela DA, Verdier N, Otero PE. Regional anesthetic techniques for the pelvic limb and abdominal wall in small animals: a review of the literature and technique description. Vet J 2018;238:27–40.
2. Gurney MA, Leece EA. Analgesia for pelvic limb surgery. A review of peripheral nerve blocks and the extradural technique. Vet Anaesth Analg 2014;41:445–58.
3. Vettorato E, Bradbrook C, Gurney M, et al. Peripheral nerve blocks of the pelvic limb in dogs: a retrospective clinical study. Vet Comp Orthop Traumatol 2012; 25(4):314–20. Germany.
4. Steinhaus ME, Rosneck J, Ahmad CS, et al. Outcomes after peripheral nerve block in hip arthroscopy. Am J Orthop (Belle Mead NJ) 2018;47. https://doi.org/10.12788/ajo.2018.0049.
5. Kessler J, Marhofer P, Hopkins PM, et al. Peripheral regional anaesthesia and outcome: lessons learned from the last 10 years. Br J Anaesth 2015;114:728–45.
6. Marhofer P, Chan VW. Ultrasound-guided regional anesthesia: current concepts and future trends. Anesth Analg 2007;104:1265–9.
7. Barrington MJ, Uda Y. Did ultrasound fulfill the promise of safety in regional anesthesia? Curr Opin Anaesthesiol 2018;31:649–55.
8. Tran DQ, Boezaart AP, Neal JM. Beyond ultrasound guidance for regional anesthesiology. Reg Anesth Pain Med 2017;42:556–63.
9. Echeverry DF, Laredo FG, Gil F, et al. Ventral ultrasound-guided suprainguinal approach to block the femoral nerve in the dog. Vet J 2012;192(3):333–7.
10. Monticelli P, Drozdzynska M, Stathopoulou T, et al. A description of a technique for ultrasound-guided lumbar plexus catheter in dogs: cadaveric study. Vet Anaesth Analg 2016;43(4):453–6.
11. Mogicato G, Layssol-Lamour C, Mahler S, et al. Anatomical and ultrasonographic study of the femoral nerve within the iliopsoas muscle in beagle dogs and cats. Vet Anaesth Analg 2015;42:425–32.
12. Portela DA, Otero PE, Briganti A, et al. Femoral nerve block: a novel psoas compartment lateral pre-iliac approach in dogs. Vet Anaesth Analg 2013;40(2):194–204.
13. Mahler SP. Ultrasound guidance to approach the femoral nerve in the iliopsoas muscle: a preliminary study in the dog. Vet Anaesth Analg 2012;39:550–4.
14. Echeverry DF, Laredo FG, Gil F, et al. Ultrasound-guided 'two-in-one' femoral and obturator nerve block in the dog: an anatomical study. Vet Anaesth Analg 2012; 39:611–7.
15. Shimada S, Shimizu M, Kishimoto M. Ultrasound-guided femoral nerve block using a ventral suprainguinal approach in healthy dogs. Vet Anaesth Analg 2017; 44:1208–15.
16. Tayari H, Tazioli G, Breghi G, et al. Ultrasound-guided femoral and obturator nerves block in the psoas compartment in dogs: anatomical and randomized clinical study. Vet Anaesth Analg 2017;44:1216–26.

17. O Cathasaigh M, Read MR, Atilla A, et al. Blood concentration of bupivacaine and duration of sensory and motor block following ultrasound-guided femoral and sciatic nerve blocks in dogs. PLoS One 2018;13:e0193400.
18. Portela DA, Otero PE, Tarragona L, et al. Combined paravertebral plexus block and parasacral sciatic block in healthy dogs. Vet Anaesth Analg 2010;37:531–41.
19. Shilo Y, Pascoe PJ, Cissell D, et al. Ultrasound-guided nerve blocks of the pelvic limb in dogs. Vet Anaesth Analg 2010;37(5):460–70.
20. Costa-Farre C, Blanch XS, Cruz JI, et al. Ultrasound guidance for the performance of sciatic and saphenous nerve blocks in dogs. Vet J 2011;187:221–4.
21. Campoy L, Bezuidenhout AJ, Gleed RD, et al. Ultrasound-guided approach for axillary brachial plexus, femoral nerve, and sciatic nerve blocks in dogs. Vet Anaesth Analg 2010;37:144–53.
22. Evans EH, de Lahunta A. Spinal nerves Miller's anatomy of the dog. 4th edition. St Louis (MO): Elsevier; 2013. p. 611–57.
23. Kinzel S, Fasselt R, Prescher A, et al. Sensory innervation of the hip joint capsule in dogs. Tierarztl Prax Ausg K Kleintiere Heimtiere 1998;26:330–5.
24. Huang CH, Hou SM, Yeh LS. The innervation of canine hip joint capsule: an anatomic study. Anat Histol Embryol 2013;42:425–31.

Epidural and Spinal Anesthesia

Manuel Martin-Flores, DVM

KEYWORDS

• Epidural • Spinal • Anesthesia • Bupivacaine • Ropivacaine

KEY POINTS

- Epidural and spinal anesthesia with a combination of local anesthetics and opioids (when available) is a commonly used technique in veterinary medicine and a safe one when practiced under strict guidelines.
- It is a valuable tool in the analgesic armamentarium and can greatly extend the ability to provide analgesia and reduce postoperative opioid requirements.
- As with all regional anesthetic techniques, clinical experience should be gained in order to practice it efficiently, and care should be taken to minimize the risks and complications associated with its use.

INTRODUCTION

Epidural anesthesia was described in dogs more than half a century ago[1] and remains one of the most commonly practiced regional anesthesia techniques. Epidural anesthesia is a versatile procedure that, through manipulations of the agents injected, their doses, and site of injection, can provide desensitization to the hind limbs, abdomen, and thorax, making it an important addition to the armamentarium for providing effective analgesia to patients. Epidural anesthesia can serve as adjuvant to general anesthetics, as the main anesthetic technique in sedated animals, or as an analgesic in awake animals requiring pain alleviation. Epidural and spinal anesthesia have been shown to be safe procedures when practiced well, to produce equal or better pain relief than systemic opioids,[2] and to blunt the increase in stress markers that follow surgery.[3] In dogs, the use of epidural anesthesia might even help reduce the risk of perianesthetic mortality. An ongoing study comparing groups of dogs with similar characteristics detected a reduced mortality of 3 per 1000 in dogs receiving an epidural, compared with 8 per 1000 cases in dogs not receiving neuraxial block (JI Redondo, 2019, data not yet published). There are no absolute indications to the use of neuraxial blockade; nevertheless, clinicians may choose to include this

Disclosures: None.

Section of Anesthesiology and Pain Medicine, Department of Clinical Sciences, College of Veterinary Medicine, Cornell University, 930 Campus Road, Ithaca, NY 14850, USA

E-mail address: martinflores@cornell.edu

technique as part of anesthetic and analgesic management to improve patient comfort and decrease the use of general anesthetics or systemic analgesics. When used for surgery of the hind limbs, epidural or spinal anesthesia may also augment muscle relaxation and facilitate surgical manipulation. Although epidural and spinal anesthesia might be used, as mentioned earlier, for a wide variety of procedures, this article focuses on the use of lumbosacral epidural and spinal anesthesia, targeted for procedures of the hind limbs in dogs.

RELEVANT ANATOMY AND TECHNIQUE

Seven cervical, 13 thoracic, 7 lumbar, 3 sacral, and a variable number of coccygeal vertebrae compose the canine and feline spinal columns. The spinal canal is formed by the sum of rings from each vertebra, and extends from the foramen magnum to approximately the sixth coccygeal vertebra. The spinal (or vertebral) canal includes the epidural space and the intrathecal structures: meninges, cerebrospinal fluid, and spinal cord. The floor of the canal is formed by the dorsal longitudinal ligament, which is attached to the vertebrae and intervertebral disks. The lateral walls are formed by the intervertebral pedicles and foramina. The vertebral laminae and the ligamentum flavum (yellow, or interarcuate ligament) compose the roof of the spinal canal (**Fig. 1**).

The spinal cord courses through most of the length of the canal, covered and enclosed by the meninges: the pia mater, the arachnoid mater, and the dura mater, ordered from innermost to outermost. The pia mater is closely adhered to the spinal cord. Cerebrospinal fluid (CSF) is found between the pia mater and the next layer, the arachnoid, in the subarachnoid space. These structures produce a physiologically active barrier that surrounds the central nervous system. The subarachnoid space extends caudally to the caudal segments of the spinal cord to form the lumbar cistern. The arachnoid is adhered to the outermost layer, the thicker dura mater. The dura mater continues caudally to form the dural sac, surrounding the cauda equina. Even more caudally, the cauda equina continues to form the filum terminale, also covered by a tapering dura mater (see **Fig. 1**). The dura is primarily composed of collagen fibers and can easily be punctured with a needle; this is a potential complication of epidural injections. In contrast, the arachnoid layer is more flexible and may deform when a needle comes in contact with it. The potential space between the dura and the

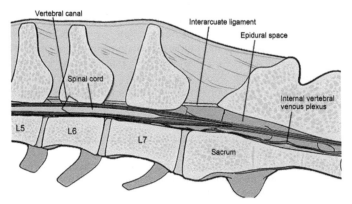

Fig. 1. The lumbosacral vertebrae, ligaments, spinal cord and meninges, and the epidural and subarachnoid spaces. (*Courtesy of* L. Campoy, LV, CertVA, Dip ECVAA, MRCVS, Ithaca, NY and Cornell University, Ithaca, NY.)

arachnoid is referred to as the subdural space. Although it is rare to perform an unintended subdural injection, it is possible.

The epidural space is an annular space delimited by the dura mater and the floor, walls, and roof of the spinal canal. At the roof, it is delimited by the ligamentum flavum. This space is larger at the lumbosacral level (and caudally), because the spinal cord and dura taper. As a consequence, the lumbosacral space is the most common location for epidural injections in small animals. In adult dogs, the dural sac typically is located between the sixth and seventh lumbar vertebrae; however, because it tapers caudally, the dural sac can also be found at the lumbosacral level (see **Fig. 1**). It may extend even more caudally in young individuals, in adult dogs of small breeds, or in cats. As a result, epidural punctures at the lumbosacral space risk perforating the dural sac and coming in contact with CSF.

The dura and arachnoid membranes also surround the spinal nerves, covering them as they exit the vertebral canal laterally through the intervertebral foramina. These layers travel with the nerve roots and blend with their connective tissue to form the nerve sheath. This region represents the site of action for epidurally administered local anesthetics, as discussed later.

The epidural space is not an empty space, nor is it a closed one; it communicates with the paravertebral space via the lateral foramina. Epidural fat is the most widespread tissue contained in the epidural space, and is found between the dura mater and the ligamentum flavum. It provides a cushion to the spinal cord, protecting it from mechanical trauma. Epidural fat is more abundant in the caudal areas of the vertebral canal, and is mainly located at the sides and roof of the epidural space. In the ventral aspect of the epidural space, the venous plexus is found. These vessels communicate with vasculature from the bones and from the spinal cord, and drain through the intervertebral foramina, in close proximity to the spinal nerves, and ultimately drain their blood to the azygos and vena cava. Increased intra-abdominal pressure may be transmitted through these veins to the epidural venous plexus, increasing their volume, which may be the case in pregnant animals, a population in which epidural anesthesia is often performed as part of the perianesthetic management of cesarean surgery. Arterial supply to the spinal cord is typically covered by the pia mater, and originates from the vertebral and segmental arteries.

In summary, the epidural space at the lumbosacral level, the target location for an epidural injection, is a small space, separated from the CSF by the meninges, and occupied by epidural fat and vessels. These characteristics should be considered when performing this technique.

MECHANISMS OF ACTION

The principal site of action of local anesthetics administered epidurally is the nerve root. Local anesthetics bathe the nerve roots as they emerge from the vertebral canal, producing conduction blockade through interaction with Na^+ channels. The hind limbs are supplied by lumbar nerves 3 to 7 (L3–L7) and the first sacral nerve (S1), and hence, the local anesthetic must be deposited in proximity to those roots for a successful block.

Local anesthetics interrupt neural conduction by preventing the conformational changes that occur in the Na^+ channels following the arrival of an action potential; the generation and transmission of action potentials are inhibited. Local anesthetics permeate through the neural membrane before interacting with the Na^+ channel. Most local anesthetics coexist in ionized and nonionized forms. It is the nonionized form that traverses the neural membrane. The agent then becomes ionized and binds to the Na^+ channel. The interaction between the local anesthetic and the Na^+ channel is best described as a state of dynamic equilibrium, in which dissociation between agent and channel may occur in between successive depolarizations.

As mentioned earlier, the site of action for epidurally administered local anesthetics is the nerve roots. Paired spinal nerves arise from spinal cord segments through the lateral foramina. Each segment gives rise to both ventral and dorsal roots; the ventral root being motor and sympathetic, and the dorsal root sensory. Both roots unite in close proximity to the foramina to form the spinal nerve, which involves both sensory and motor components. Studies in humans show that dorsal roots often divide into 2 or 3 different bundles on exiting the spinal cord, and that those bundles may further separate into several different fascicles.[4,5] As a result, the dorsal, multifascicular root presents a larger surface area for local anesthetic uptake than the smaller, single, ventral root. This difference may favor access and uptake of the local anesthetic into the dorsal, sensory root, and may be at least in part responsible for the development of selective sensory blockade.

The uptake of local anesthetics into each nerve root determines the effects produced during epidural anesthesia. This uptake depends primarily on the concentration of the local anesthetic in the epidural space at the perineural level (or the CSF in the case of spinal anesthesia). The concentration of local anesthetic is determined primarily by the concentration of the agent selected, and is affected by the distribution of the solution injected; a gradient of concentration occurs, with the highest concentration found at the site of injection. Direct assessment of the distribution (or extent) of epidural anesthesia is not an easy task, because it requires the quantification of local anesthetic concentration at the site of action. A clinically useful and more practical alternative is to consider dermatomes as sensory extensions of the spinal cord segments and test sensitivity at that level. Hence, the qualitative assessment of sensory function (eg, by pinprick) is often used to assess local anesthetic distribution and the extent of blockade.[6]

When local anesthetics are injected at the level of the lumbosacral space, the solution disperses both cranially and caudally. In addition, the solution may also distribute laterally and exit through the foramina. The distribution of local anesthetic determines the extent of block, and it is largely affected by the volume injected.[6,7] As mentioned earlier, the pelvic limb is innervated by spinal nerves arising from L3 to S1, and hence, distribution of the epidural block needs not surpass those levels. An unnecessarily large distribution of local anesthetic (cephalad extent) does not provide additional analgesia to the pelvic limb and increases the risk of sympathetic block and its associated decrease in arterial pressure. Evidence in humans suggests that the total dose of local anesthetic administered, and not just the volume, can also affect the distribution of the epidural blockade.[8,9] Although there is no substantial evidence to corroborate this assertion in dogs, it is possible that, when using an equal volume, concentrated solutions may result in larger distribution of the epidural blockade.

Although it may be intuitive that a fast epidural injection could result in wider distribution of block, this hypothesis has not been confirmed in dogs. In people, rapid injections result in higher increases in epidural pressure and an initial increase in the distribution of sensory blockade.[10,11] However, the ultimate distribution of sensory blockade is not affected. In dogs, distribution of sensory blockade and distribution of injectate were not affected by doubling the speed of injection, but higher epidural pressures were reached when a faster speed was used.[12] High epidural pressure may result in direct injury to the spinal cord or nerves, or may interfere with perfusion. Hence, despite the lack of evidence associating injection speed with distribution of the injectate, it is recommended to exert caution during epidural injections and avoid abrupt increases in epidural pressure.

INDICATIONS AND TECHNIQUE

Epidural and spinal anesthesia can be performed in sedated or anesthetized dogs, whether it is to provide pain relief in traumatized animals, after a surgical procedure, or for its anesthetic-sparing effects during surgery. Whether placed under sedation or general anesthesia, basic standards for sedation and anesthesia are to be followed. In all cases, an intravenous catheter should be placed, and vital signs, such as an electrocardiogram, pulse-oximetry (Spo_2), and/or arterial blood pressure, should be monitored. In addition, materials to secure the airway (including suction) and provide oxygen should be guaranteed. With these provisions, depth of sedation could be safely tailored with short-acting intravenous agents, such as propofol, so that the procedure can be tolerated comfortably by the dog. Deep sedation or general anesthesia might be required in dogs with trauma. When placed presurgically, epidural injections are most often performed under general anesthesia.

In sedated animals, the area of puncture can be desensitized by infiltration with lidocaine. This desensitization is unnecessary in dogs under general anesthesia. Dogs may be positioned in sternal or lateral recumbency, depending on the preferences of the operator and the dog's medical condition, such as the presence of pelvic or pelvic-limb fractures. It is typically preferred to perform epidural injections with the animal in sternal recumbency, because it favors recognition of anatomic landmarks. In either recumbency, it is helpful to flex the spine by placing the hind limbs in a forward position, because this widens the distance between spinous processes.[13,14]

The lumbosacral space is identified through palpation of the spinous processes; care should be taken to adequately palpate L6, L7, and S1, because L7 might be difficult to identify in some dogs because of the lower height of its spinous process. An area over the lumbosacral space should be clipped and surgically scrubbed, with sufficient margins to allow placement of a fenestrated sterile drape. Sterile gloves should always be used when performing this procedure (**Fig. 2**).

Tuohy needles are recommended for epidural injections; these needles have external centimeter markings that indicate depth of the puncture. Tuohy needles are typically winged, allowing secure handling of the needle as the relatively blunt bevel penetrates the different tissues. The bevel is not only blunt but also curved forward, which allows the insertion of a catheter should one be used and provides a better tactile feedback, improving the detection of the spinous ligaments as the needle is advanced. The lack of sharpness of the bevel may also help prevent accidental spinal punctures. Lastly, these needles are provided with an internal mandrel or stylet that prevents obstructions within the lumen with tissue as the needle is advanced (**Fig. 3**).

With the dog in sternal recumbency, and after having identified the appropriate anatomic landmarks (lumbosacral space), the needle is slowly inserted perpendicularly to the skin, approximately halfway between the L7 and S1 processes. Tuohy needles are held by the wings, and the operator supports the hands over the skin of the dog, as shown in **Fig. 3**. This technique provides stability and prevents sudden and unintended deep insertions of the needle as each tissue layer is penetrated. The needle is advanced through the skin, subcutaneous tissue, and into the interspinous ligament (clinical tip: once the needle is advanced into the interspinous ligament, it will remain firmly implanted in it, and will remain vertical even if not held. If the needle falls when not held, it is likely superficial or lateral to this ligament). As the needle is advanced further, the interarcuate ligament is punctured and the epidural space

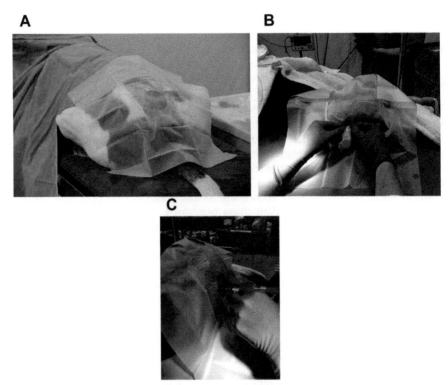

Fig. 2. Two dogs placed in (*A*) ventral and (*B & C*) lateral recumbency during an epidural injection. Sterile gloves are used and fenestrated drapes are placed over the skin after the lumbosacral space is clipped and surgically scrubbed. (**Fig. 2**A, *Courtesy of* L. Campoy, LV, CertVA, Dip ECVAA, MRCVS, Ithaca, NY and Cornell University, Ithaca, NY.)

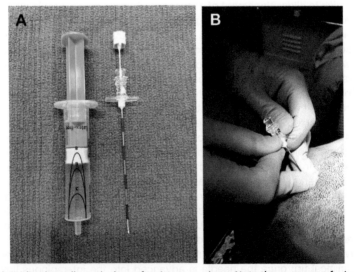

Fig. 3. (*A*) Epidural needle and a loss-of-resistance syringe. Note the presence of wings, which allow easier manipulation, marked shaft, and a partially removed mandrel. (*B*) Epidural injection using a Tuohy needle. Note that the operators hold the needle by the wings, and support their hands over the lumbar region of the dog, close to the puncture site.

accessed. A distinctive change in resistance to the insertion of the needle is typically appreciated (not typically appreciated with sharp, spinal, or hypodermic needles).

There are 2 main techniques to identify the correct (epidural) location of the tip of the needle: the loss of resistance (LOR), as described by its name, is based on the sensation of resistance to injection as the epidural needle traverses the different tissue layers; a specifically designed syringe is used. Attempts to inject either air or saline are made (either pulsatile or continuous) during insertion of the epidural needle. Resistance to injection is high while the needle is embedded in the ligaments, and it is suddenly lost when the tip of the needle punctures the interarcuate ligament and enters the epidural space. False-positives (LOR) might occur if the needle is placed oblique as the tip of the needle exits the ligament. False-negatives (no LOR) might occur if the lumen of needle is obstructed with tissue as the needle is advanced. When LOR is detected, injection should be immediately stopped, especially when air is used, because epidural air might interfere with an even distribution of the injectate, or contribute to compression of the spinal cord.

The hanging drop method is performed by applying a solution (typically normal saline or local anesthetic) into the hub of the needle, once the stylet is removed. The drop can be observed to enter the needle hub when the tip of the needle penetrates the interarcuate ligament. This technique works best when used with the animal in sternal recumbency.[15]

Other techniques have also been described to assist in confirming correct location of the epidural needle. Electrolocation has been described in dogs, and it is based on the positive motor response to nerve stimulation; as the needle approximates the spinal cord, the required stimulus to elicit a response is reduced. When performed at the lumbosacral space, a current of 0.3 mA (pulse with 0.1 millisecond) positively elicits motor responses if the tip of the needle is located in the epidural space.[16] Ultrasonography can also be used to help confirm the correct placement of the epidural needle. Ultrasonography can be used to identify anatomic landmarks and visualize the epidural space,[17] especially in obese dogs, in which it is otherwise difficult to palpate anatomic landmarks, and can also be used to observe the passage of fluid as the injection is performed.

On reaching the epidural space, insertion of the needle stops; the hub is then examined for the presence of blood or CSF, either being a potential complication at the lumbosacral space. If neither fluid is encountered, the syringe with the local anesthetic or analgesic solution is attached to the needle, either directly or via a short extension line. Extension lines allow some manipulation and decrease the chances of inadvertent movement of the needle. Once the syringe is attached, the operator should aspirate and again examine the absence of blood or CSF. Evidence of either fluid should prevent the operator from injecting the solution and avoid either a spinal anesthesia overdose or local anesthesia toxicity from intravascular injection. If no complications are encountered, the epidural injection is performed slowly and with the absence of resistance.

SACROCOCCYGEAL EPIDURAL INJECTION

The sacrococcygeal (SC) space can also be used for epidural injections. The space can be recognized through palpation of anatomic landmarks, and location of the needle can be confirmed as described earlier. The anatomic structures are smaller at this level and hence correct positioning of the needle might be more difficult to identify. Smaller structures (eg, a thinner interarcuate ligament) may give the operator less feedback through the needle regarding its position, which is further complicated by the different angle at which the puncture is performed (typically 45° to the skin). However, the risk of a spinal puncture is minimized, this being likely the most important advantage of this approach. A recent study suggests that the volume of injection needs not be altered if a lumbosacral injection is replaced by the SC approach, facilitating the implementation of this technique into clinical practice.[18]

EPIDURAL CATHETER

Touhy needles allow the passage of an epidural catheter, which can be left in situ and used for repeated injections or infusions of different solutions. The placement of an epidural catheter further increases the versatility of this technique, and not only makes possible the prolongation of effects by administering more doses but also allows titration of the dose of injections until a desired effect is reached.

Once the insertion of the Touhy needle is completed, the epidural catheter is advanced into the hub of the needle, facilitated with an adapter provided in the continual epidural kit. While the catheter is advanced into the needle, resistance is perceived as the tip of the catheter reaches the bevel of the needle. This resistance is lost as the catheter exits the needle, and no further resistance is typically encountered. The catheters are marked so that the depth of insertion can be measured. Ideally, the tip of the catheter is placed in close proximity to the target nerve roots. When targeting the hind limbs, the injected solution should bathe the roots between L3 and S1 and, hence, the tip of the catheter should be position within that segment. Excessive threading of the catheter results in blockade outside the area of interest. The operator should also consider that the catheter may not follow a direct path while being advanced; lateralization and coiling are possible. It is also recommended that the catheter is only advanced forward and not retrieved back while being inserted through the needle, because the backward passage through the bevel may cut the catheter.

Once the catheter is advanced to its desired length, the epidural needle is removed while the catheter is held in place. An injection adapter and a filter are placed in the outer end of the catheter. The catheter is then secured with adhesive dressing. The operator may choose to tunnel the catheter a short distance to provide additional fixation. Catheters should also be examined for the presence of CSF or blood, which may not have been apparent during insertion of the needle. If the catheter is placed for intraoperative use, the distal end of the catheter can be located cranially so that it can be accessed during surgery. For postoperative use, the catheter is typically coiled over the lumbosacral space, covered with extra adhesive dressing, and labeled. Injections through the catheter are characterized by a high resistance, caused by the length and small diameter of the catheter (**Fig. 4**).

EPIDURAL DOSING: VOLUMES AND AGENTS

The most common method to dose local anesthetics for epidural injection is based on the relationship between volume of injectate and weight of the patient (mL/kg). An alternative approach is to calculate the volume of epidural solution based on the length of the spine, measured from occipital condyle to first coccygeal vertebra (mL/cm). When targeting the hind limbs, small volumes of injections are needed given the proximity of the injection site and the target nerve roots. It is unclear whether any method is superior. A volume of 0.2 mL/kg has been reported to reach the L1 segment, and hence should be sufficient for blockade of the hind limbs.[6,19] It is possible that volumes between 0.15 and 0.2 mL/kg provide sufficient distribution for anesthesia

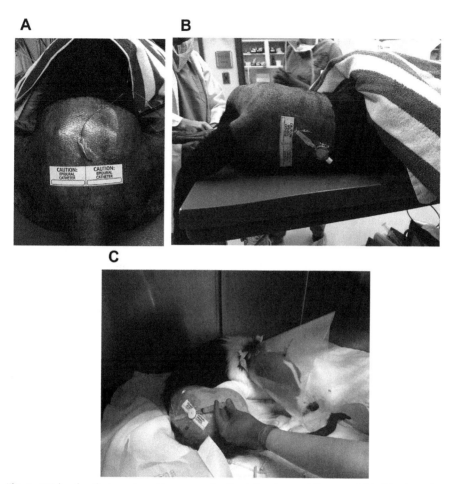

Fig. 4. Epidural catheters placed in an anesthetized dog from a (*A*) top and (*B*) side view: the catheter is tunneled under the skin and covered by a transparent adhesive sterile drape. The catheter is extended cranially to allow access by the anesthesia provider during surgery if redosing is necessary. The catheter is then fixed in place for use in the postoperative period. (*C*) An epidural catheter being used to redose postoperative in a dog.

of these segments. When the length of the spine is used to guide dosing, a volume of 0.05 mL/cm has been suggested for block of the caudal third of the spine.[20] When these two dosing regimens were compared, the total calculated volume was slightly smaller when milliliters per centimeter was used; however, no comparisons on the efficacy of each method have been reported.[21]

Duration and depth of blockade are affected by the agent of choice, the concentration of that agent, and the use of adjuvants. Lidocaine and bupivacaine are likely the most commonly used agents, with ropivacaine also gaining popularity. A summary of the characteristics of these drugs is given in **Table 1**; as a general rule, lidocaine acts faster and for a shorter time than bupivacaine or ropivacaine. Concentrated solutions of local anesthetics (eg, bupivacaine 0.5% or lidocaine 2%) result in complete sensory block accompanied with hind-limb paralysis. Solutions of lower concentration (eg, bupivacaine ≤0.25% or lidocaine ≤1%) may

Table 1
Short-acting and long-acting local anesthetics used commonly for epidural anesthesia in dogs and cats

Agent	Onset (min)	Approximate Duration (h)
Lidocaine 2%	5	2–4
Bupivacaine 0.5%	10	4–6
Ropivacaine 0.5%	10	4–6

Only solutions free of preservative should be used for this purpose

provide incomplete sensory function but preserve motor function (even if incomplete). The agent and concentration should be selected with considerations of the length and invasiveness of the procedure, and the desired postoperative effects. A sequence of varying concentrations may be used when an epidural catheter is placed. For example, a concentrated local anesthetic is administered preoperatively to provide complete sensory block during surgery. The concurrent motor block provides muscle relaxation during surgery, which may improve the operating field. Postoperatively, lower concentrations of local anesthetics are administered to prolong analgesia while retaining motor function. This author commonly uses bupivacaine (or ropivacaine) 0.5% before surgery, followed by lower concentrations (0.1%–0.2%) postoperatively (see **Table 1**).

ADJUVANTS

Several agents have been used epidurally in combination with local anesthetics, including and not restricted to opioids, alpha$_2$-agonists, ketamine, and neostigmine; opioids are the most commonly used in veterinary medicine. Opioids are added to local anesthetics to either augment the efficacy of analgesia or to prolong the duration of analgesia, especially in the postoperative period. The addition of opioids may reduce the dose of local anesthetic and reduce its associated motor effects. Epidural opioids must traverse the meninges in order to reach their target receptors: opioid receptors in the dorsal horn of the spinal cord. However, once deposited in the epidural space, the agents may diffuse through meninges following a concentration gradient, or redistribute into the epidural fat. Agents with high liposolubility preferentially redistribute into epidural fat, making them unavailable to traverse the meninges and reach the CSF and more prone to be cleared via capillaries. Epidural opioids may then produce their analgesic effects by 2 mechanisms: spinal analgesia occurs by the interaction with opioid receptors in the dorsal horn of the spinal cord, or supraspinal analgesia, which occurs by interactions with opioid receptors in the brainstem. This outcome is the result of cephalad distribution within the CSF or by systemic absorption from the epidural space. A combination of both mechanisms typically occurs, but the extent of whichever mechanism is dominating is affected by the characteristics of each agent. Spinal analgesia is the predominant mechanism of action for hydrophilic agents such as morphine. The mechanism of action for lipophilic agents such as fentanyl is less clear. Evidence in humans shows that, when fentanyl is infused epidurally, no differences in terms of analgesia or side effects are found with those patients receiving an equal infusion of intravenous fentanyl, suggesting that the effects observed are the result of supraspinal analgesia.[22] However, a different study compared the effects of epidural fentanyl administered either as a bolus or an infusion.[23] That study found that bolus administration resulted in segmental (spinal) analgesia, whereas the infusion resulted in nonsegmental (supraspinal) analgesia. These findings suggest that a bolus of fentanyl may create a gradient of concentration that results in the passage of fentanyl to the dorsal horn of the spinal cord to produce segmental analgesia. Such gradient may not take place during infusions of this drug, and hence segmental analgesia may not occur. These results support the clinical observation that the addition of fentanyl to local anesthetics does result in enhanced segmental block. The ultimate result of epidural administration of opioids is effective analgesia with lower doses and fewer side effects (or of lower magnitude) than those observed from systemic administration of the same agents. Nonetheless, and as mentioned earlier, systemic absorption of epidurally administered opioids occurs, and effects (and side effects) arising from systemic absorption are also observed.

The combination of either lidocaine or bupivacaine with morphine has been extensively used in veterinary medicine. Owing to its characteristics, morphine provides long-lasting analgesia that extends beyond that provided by the combined application of bupivacaine, and produces no motor blockade.[19,24] More recently, other agents have been introduced to practice. Epidural fentanyl is commonly used in humans to augment the sensory block produce by local anesthetics and has been used clinically in dogs.[25,26] Methadone is also administered epidurally in dogs, and it was shown to decrease the minimum alveolar concentration of isoflurane for a longer time than an equal intravenous dose.[27] Buprenorphine has recently been reported for epidural use in dogs, with effects apparently similar to those of morphine.[28] A list of several opioids used epidurally in small animals can be found in **Table 2**.

EXTENDED DELIVERY OF EPIDURAL AGENTS THROUGH A CATHETER

The delivery of epidural anesthetics can be extended by either repeating doses or continuously infusing a solution via an epidural catheter. There is little evidence in dogs to guide the use of repeated injections or epidural infusions of local anesthetics. Empirically, local anesthetics are repeated at an interval that represents the expected duration of that agent, or, preferentially, guided by the frequent assessment of pain on the patient by the use of validated pain score systems (eg, the Glasgow Composite Pain Scale). When the administration of epidural anesthesia is to be extended, the concentration of the local anesthetic may be reduced over time to promote earlier recovery of motor function. It is also expected that the degree of pain will decrease with time and so would the requirements of analgesics. Also empirically, the volume injected through the catheter for subsequent redosing via repeated boluses might be similar or slightly less than the one injected initially. The volume might need to be reduced depending on the location of the tip of the catheter. Also empirically, infusions

Table 2		
Opioids used commonly in combination with local anesthetics during epidural anesthesia in dogs and cats		
Agent	**Dose**	**Approximate Duration (h)**
Morphine	0.1 mg/kg	6–24
Fentanyl	2–5 μg/mL of solution Or 2–5 μg/kg[a]	3–5
Buprenorphine	4 μg/kg	12–24

It is recommended that only solutions free of preservatives be used for this purpose.
[a] Note that fentanyl has been used with different dosing strategies that are not interchangeable.

of local anesthetics might be set initially to deliver a calculated bolus dose divided over the time of expected effects. For example, if a bolus of 0.2 mL/kg is expected to provide analgesia for 6 hours, that same volume may be infused over that time interval. Infusions require close monitoring of the patient to detect either underdosing or overdosing. Because a small volume is delivered at a given time during an infusion, it is important that the tip of the catheter is situated in close proximity to the target nerve roots. By opposition, injection of larger boluses through a catheter may help overcome inaccurate locations of the catheter (clinical tip: the author prefers to perform the first bolus injection through the needle, before placement of the catheter. The injection helps open the epidural space, which may then facilitate catheter placement).

SIDE EFFECTS AND COMPLICATIONS OF EPIDURAL ANESTHESIA

Puncture of a vessel or the dural sac is a common complication during epidural anesthesia, especially when the lumbosacral space is targeted (**Fig. 5**). Careful observation of the needle hub and aspiration are recommended to avoid the inadvertent injection into those spaces. An epidural dose injected into the CSF results in excessive distribution of block with its associated sympathetic block (which may include the cardioaccelerator nerves), total spinal anesthesia, or death. Unintended intravenous injection may result in local anesthetic toxicity, the consequences of which depend on the agent and dose used. Arterial hypotension resulting from sympathetic blockade should always be considered a potential complication from the use of epidural local anesthetics; however, it is unlikely to occur when low volumes are injected. Neural

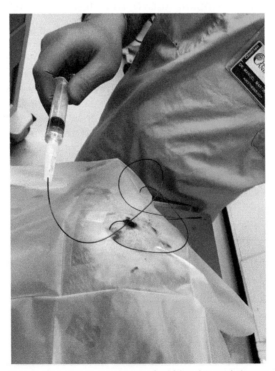

Fig. 5. Epidural catheter placed in a dog. Note that blood is withdrawn during aspiration, before the injection of the local anesthetic. No blood was noted during aspiration when the puncture was performed.

toxicity may result when agents with untested agents are used, including preserva-tives. Hence, only preservative-free solutions, or doses labeled as approved for epidural use, should be used. A hematoma may result from the accidental puncture of a vessel. Typically, coagulation limits the extent of the hematoma. However, in animals with coagulopathy, a large mass may form from the hemorrhage, which could compress neural structures; this technique is contraindicated when coagulation is impaired. Infections at the site of injection also preclude the use of epidurals. Cases of discospondylitis following epidural injections have been reported in dogs.[29,30]

SUMMARY

Epidural and spinal anesthesia with a combination of local anesthetics and opioids (when available) is a commonly used technique in veterinary medicine and a safe one when practiced under strict guidelines. It is a valuable tool in the analgesic arma-mentarium that can greatly extend the ability to provide analgesia and reduce postop-erative opioid requirements. As with all regional anesthetic techniques, clinical experience should be gained in order to practice it efficiently, and care should be taken to minimize the risks and complications associated with its use.

REFERENCES

1. Bone JK, Peck JG. Epidural anesthesia in dogs. J Am Vet Med Assoc 1956;128: 236–8.
2. Hoelzler MG, Harvey RC, Lidbetter DA, et al. Comparison of perioperative anal-gesic protocols for dogs undergoing tibial plateau leveling osteotomy. Vet Surg 2005;34:337–44.
3. Romano M, Portela DA, Breghi G, et al. Stress-related biomarkers in dogs admin-istered regional anaesthesia or fentanyl for analgesia during stifle surgery. Vet Anaesth Analg 2016;43:44–54.
4. Hogan Q. Size of human lower thoracic and lumbosacral nerve roots. Anesthesi-ology 1996;85:37–42.
5. Hogan Q, Toth J. Anatomy of soft tissues of the spinal canal. Reg Anesth Pain Med 1999;24:303–10.
6. Freire CD, Torres ML, Fantoni DT, et al. Bupivacaine 0.25% and methylene blue spread with epidural anesthesia in dog. Vet Anaesth Analg 2010;37:63–9.
7. Duke T, Caulkett NA, Ball SD, et al. Comparative analgesic and cardiopulmonary effects of epidural bupivacaine and ropivacaine in conscious dogs. Vet Anaesth Analg 2000;27:102–3.
8. Nakayama M, Yamamoto J, Ichinose H, et al. Effects of volume and concentration of lidocaine on epidural anaesthesia in pregnant females. Eur J Anaesthesiol 2002;19:808–11.
9. Sakura S, Sumi M, Kushizaki H, et al. Concentration of lidocaine affects intensity of sensory block during lumbar epidural anesthesia. Anesth Analg 1999;88: 123–7.
10. Griffiths RB, Horton WA, Jones IG, et al. Speed of injection and spread of bupi-vacaine in the epidural space. Anaesthesia 1987;42:160–3.
11. Kanai A, Suzuki A, Hoka S. Rapid injection of epidural mepivacaine speeds the onset of nerve blockade. Can J Anaesth 2005;52:281–4.
12. Son WG, Jang M, Yoon J, et al. The effect of epidural injection speed on epidural pressure and distribution of solution in anesthetized dogs. Vet Anaesth Analg 2014;41:526–33.

13. Panti A, Greenhalgh SN, Longo M, et al. The effect of recumbency and hindlimb position on the lumbosacral interlaminar distance in dogs: a cadaveric computed tomography study. Vet Anaesth Analg 2018;45:802–10.
14. Puggioni A, Arnett R, Clegg T, et al. Influence of patient positioning on the l5-l6 mid-laminar distance. Vet Radiol Ultrasound 2006;47:449–52.
15. Naganobu K, Hagio M. The effect of body position on the 'hanging drop' method for identifying the extradural space in anaesthetized dogs. Vet Anaesth Analg 2007;34:59–62.
16. Garcia-Pereira FL, Hauptman J, Shih AC, et al. Evaluation of electric neurostimulation to confirm correct placement of lumbosacral epidural injections in dogs. Am J Vet Res 2010;71:157–60.
17. Liotta A, Busoni V, Carrozzo MV, et al. Feasibility of ultrasound-guided epidural access at the lumbo-sacral space in dogs. Vet Radiol Ultrasound 2015;56:220–8.
18. Vesovski S, Makara M, Martinez-Taboada F. Computer tomographic comparison of cranial spread of contrast in lumbosacral and sacrococcygeal epidural injections in dog cadavers. Vet Anaesth Analg 2019;46:510–5.
19. Campoy L, Martin-Flores M, Ludders JW, et al. Comparison of bupivacaine femoral and sciatic nerve block versus bupivacaine and morphine epidural for stifle surgery in dogs. Vet Anaesth Analg 2012;39:91–8.
20. Otero P, Tarragona L, Ceballos M, et al. Epidural cephalic spread of a local anesthetic in dogs: a mathematical model using the column length. Proceedings of the 10th World Congress of Veterinary Anaesthesia. Glasgow, UK, August 31 - September 4, 2009.
21. Valverde A, Skelding A. Comparison of calculated lumbosacral epidural volumes of injectate using a dose regimen based on body weight versus length of the vertebral column in dogs. Vet Anaesth Analg 2019;46:135–40.
22. Loper KA, Ready LB, Downey M, et al. Epidural and intravenous fentanyl infusions are clinically equivalent after knee surgery. Anesth Analg 1990;70:72–5.
23. Ginosar Y, Riley ET, Angst MS. The site of action of epidural fentanyl in humans: the difference between infusion and bolus administration. Anesth Analg 2003;97:1428–38.
24. Valverde A, Dyson DH, McDonell WN. Epidural morphine reduces halothane MAC in the dog. Can J Anaesth 1989;36:629–32.
25. Diniz MS, Kanashiro GP, Bernardi CA, et al. Extradural anesthesia with lidocaine combined with fentanyl or methadone to ovariohisterectomy in dogs. Acta Cir Bras 2013;28:531–6.
26. Saritas ZK, Saritas TB, Pamuk K, et al. Comparison of the effects of lidocaine and fentanyl in epidural anesthesia in dogs. Bratisl Lek Listy 2014;115:508–13.
27. Campagnol D, Teixeira-Neto FJ, Peccinini RG, et al. Comparison of the effects of epidural or intravenous methadone on the minimum alveolar concentration of isoflurane in dogs. Vet J 2012;192:311–5.
28. Bartel AK, Campoy L, Martin-Flores M, et al. Comparison of bupivacaine and dexmedetomidine femoral and sciatic nerve blocks with bupivacaine and buprenorphine epidural injection for stifle arthroplasty in dogs. Vet Anaesth Analg 2016;43:435–43.
29. MacFarlane PD, Iff I. Discospondylitis in a dog after attempted extradural injection. Vet Anaesth Analg 2011;38:272–3.
30. Remedios AM, Wagner R, Caulkett NA, et al. Epidural abscess and discospondylitis in a dog after administration of a lumbosacral epidural analgesic. Can Vet J 1996;37:106–7.

Local Anesthetics
Pharmacology and Special Preparations

Michele Barletta, DVM, MS, PhD*, Rachel Reed, DVM

KEYWORDS

- Clinical use • Exparel • Lidocaine patch • Liposomal bupivacaine
- Local anesthetics • Nocita • Pharmacology

KEY POINTS

- Local anesthetics are the only drugs that can fully block nociception by blocking the action potentials within neurons via inhibition of voltage-gated sodium channels.
- They are weak bases, with a molecular weight ranging from 220 to 288 Da.
- Lidocaine can be administered systemically to provide analgesia, antiinflammatory effects, antiarrhythmic effects, and reduction in inhalant anesthetic requirements, and to enhance gastrointestinal motility and free-radical scavenging.
- Lidocaine patches are used in veterinary medicine for postoperative pain; however, published data do not support their use.
- Liposomal bupivacaine is an extended-release formulation that can provide pain relief up to 72 hours after administration.

INTRODUCTION

Local anesthetics are the only class of drugs that can fully block nociceptive impulses from reaching the cerebral cortex and, thus, they represent the only means of completely preventing patient perception of a nociceptive stimulus. Since their introduction in the late 1800s, use of local anesthetics has continuously increased in popularity. Today, this class of drugs is used routinely for peripheral nerve blockade, neuraxial anesthesia, and even as intravenous infusions, affording many benefits to the recipient.

History

The first report of local anesthetic use in the literature occurred in 1884 when Carl Köller published on the use of cocaine to desensitize the cornea facilitating ophthalmic

Disclosure Statement: The authors have nothing to disclose.
Department of Large Animal Medicine, College of Veterinary Medicine, University of Georgia, 2200 College Station Road, Athens, GA 30602, USA
* Corresponding author.
E-mail address: mbarlett@uga.edu

procedures. Over the following years, the use of cocaine rapidly expanded for both medical and recreational use. Indeed, cocaine was an ingredient in the soda product Coca Cola until 1903. The toxic effects of cocaine quickly became evident and the search for a less toxic local anesthetic began.[1] In 1904, procaine was patented by Einhorn,[2] followed by tetracaine. Both drugs were found to have limited clinical utility and were associated with toxicity. In 1948, synthesis of lidocaine brought a more stable and less toxic local anesthetic.[3] Since that time, the use of lidocaine for local anesthesia and as an intravenous infusion has become a popular means of providing analgesia. In the following years, additional local anesthetics were synthesized, all with varying characteristics, affording differences in onset time, duration of action, and toxicity.

PHYSICAL PROPERTIES

Local anesthetics are weak bases with a pKa (dissociation constant) of 7.5 to 8.5, and are divided into 2 categories based on their structure: aminoamides or aminoesters. The general structure of all agents consists of an aromatic group connected to a tertiary amine via an amide linkage (aminoamide) or an ester linkage (aminoester).

Four physicochemical properties determine the activity of local anesthetic agents: molecular weight (MW), pKa, lipid solubility, and degree of protein binding.

Ranging from 220 to 288 Da, the MW is inversely related to the ability of the local anesthetic to diffuse through tissue. Just as changes in MW are caused by differing substitutions on the aromatic group and tertiary amine, changes in MW are generally also associated with changes in pKa and lipid solubility.[4]

As weak bases, local anesthetics equilibrate into ionized and nonionized molecules within the body in accordance with their pKa. By definition, the pKa is the pH at which the drug is at equilibrium with 50% in the ionized form and 50% in the nonionized form. The local anesthetic binding site on the sodium channel is within the cell and the drug must diffuse into the target neuron cell body to have an effect. It is the nonionized form of the drug that can easily cross the cell membrane[5] and, once inside the cell, a new equilibrium is established and the ionized (active) form of the drug can take effect.[6] In general, agents with a low pKa will have a rapid onset of action due to a lower degree of ionization at physiologic pH and agents with a high pKa will have a slower onset of action due to the greater degree of ionization at physiologic pH.

The structure of the aromatic group is the main determinant of the agent's solubility. The degree of solubility is extremely important because it determines the potency[6] and duration of action of the agent.[7] Agents with low lipid solubility have low potency and a shorter duration of action. Agents with high lipid solubility tend to be more potent and afford a longer duration of action. Lipid solubility also affects onset of action in that highly lipid soluble agents are more likely to be sequestered in myelin, slowing the arrival of the agent at the neuronal membrane and prolonging the onset of action.

The degree of protein binding determines the free fraction of drug available to bind to the target receptors and cause an effect. In general, agents that are highly protein bound are associated with a longer duration of action.[8]

MECHANISM OF ACTION

Local anesthetic agents block action potentials within neurons via inhibition of voltage-gated sodium channels. Voltage-gated sodium channels exist in 3 potential conformations: open, closed, and inactive. While resting, the channel is in the closed state and, when depolarization occurs, the channel opens and subsequently enters an inactive state, facilitating repolarization of the nerve cell membrane.[9,10] With the local anesthetic bound to the ion channel, the inactive states of the sodium channel become favored, thus inhibiting the movement of action potentials along affected nerve fibers. When a local anesthetic is present within the cell, the open and inactive states of the sodium channel provide the most favorable conditions for local anesthetic binding. This means that stimulation of nerve fibers facilitates onset of local anesthetic effect.[11,12] This phenomenon is termed frequency-dependent blockade.

PHARMACOKINETICS

Absorption of local anesthetics from the site of administration is determined by lipid solubility, vascularity of the injection site, and whether or not a vasoconstrictor (ie, epinephrine) is incorporated into the local anesthetic solution. Agents with higher lipid solubility will be less rapidly absorbed with a lower maximum plasma concentration (Cmax) and longer time to Cmax (Tmax). An opposite effect is observed when the agent is deposited into highly vascular areas, with a higher Cmax and shorter Tmax associated with the close proximity to vessels. The use of a vasoconstricting agent decreases the systemic absorption of the local anesthetic, which remains within the injection site for a longer period of time. However, care should be taken when incorporating a vasoconstricting agent because ischemic injury can result, especially if used in a body extremity. Other factors that may positively influence the achieved Cmax include use of a higher dose, the cardiac output of the patient, and vasodilation in the region associated with nerve blockade.[4]

Volume of distribution of local anesthetics mainly depends on the structure of the agent. Aminoamides are widely distributed, whereas the rapidly metabolized amino-esters have a much smaller volume of distribution. First-pass pulmonary uptake of aminoamides can significantly decrease the plasma concentration of drug after administration, especially in agents with high lipid solubility and a low pKa.[4]

Aminoamide local anesthetics are metabolized primarily by cytochrome P450 enzymes in the liver and eliminated by the kidneys.[4] Of note, lidocaine is metabolized to the active metabolite monoethylglycinexylidide, having approximately 70% of the activity of the parent molecule.[4,13] Aminoesters are degraded by cholinesterases in the plasma and in the liver, with metabolites rapidly excreted via the kidneys, affording the small volume of distribution stated previously.[14]

CLINICAL USE

Local anesthetic agents are most commonly used clinically to provide analgesia via neural blockade. This can be achieved via several different techniques, including injection in tissue surrounding the injury, perineural injection proximal to the site of injury, epidural or spinal administration, or injection into cavities such as the pleural space (these are discussed in detail in subsequent articles of this issue). Local anesthetic techniques provide blockade of nociceptive action potentials in sensory nerve fibers. As such, they are the only means of completely eliminating pain without inducing unconsciousness.

Often, clinicians will choose to mix local anesthetics to take advantage of the different characteristics of the agents (**Table 1**), such as mixing an agent with a rapid onset of action (ie, lidocaine) with an agent that has a long duration of action (ie, bupivacaine). However, a large body of research has revealed that this strategy does not in fact afford both characteristics to the block. Conversely, the opposite may occur with onset of blockade not significantly hastened and the duration of action may actually be decreased. This is likely due to alteration in the pKa and concentration of the agents by mixing the 2 together.[15–18] Based on the overwhelming evidence indicating a lack of

Table 1
Pharmacodynamic characteristics of the commonly used local anesthetic agents

Drug	Onset of Action (min)	Duration of Action (h)	Maximum Dose (mg/kg)	Notes
Aminoamides				
Lidocaine	5–10	1–1.5	Canine: 6–10 Feline: 3–5	Can be administered intravenously
Mepivacaine	5–10	1.5–2	Canine: 5–6 Feline: 2–3	—
Bupivacaine	20–30	3–10	Canine: 2 Feline: 1–1.5	—
Levobupivacaine	20–30	3–10	Canine: 2 Feline: 1–1.5	Less cardiotoxic than bupivacaine
Ropivacaine	20–30	3–6	Canine: 3 Feline: 1.5	—
Aminoesters				
Procaine	5–10	0.5–1	2–4	May cause allergic reactions due to production of PABA

Abbreviation: PABA, paraaminobenzoic acid.

advantage in mixing local anesthetics, it is currently recommended to use only 1 agent at a time.

The ideal local anesthetic agent would provide a longer duration of action than the commonly used agents today, sparing the patient from the acute pain suffered directly after insult to the tissues. Currently used strategies to circumvent this issue are techniques such as wound soaker catheters, epidural catheters, and perineural catheters. These modalities allow for multiple administrations or a constant rate infusion of the drug in the area. However, these techniques come with their own disadvantages, including increased cost, high technical skill, maintenance of the catheter, and risk of infection. One solution to this problem was proposed with the use of lidocaine patches in the area around tissue injury, providing a prolonged source of local anesthetic administered transdermally. Another recently available product, a liposome encapsulated formulation of bupivacaine (Nocita), has become available, boasting a 72-hour duration of action (see later discussion of lidocaine patches and Nocita).

Systemic Lidocaine Administration

Lidocaine is commonly administered systemically via intravenous infusion and has many beneficial effects, including analgesia, antiinflammatory effects, antiarrhythmic effects, reduction in inhalant anesthetic requirements, enhanced gastrointestinal (GI) motility, and free-radical scavenging activity. The exact mechanism of the analgesic effect is unknown but is most likely associated with inhibition of neural sodium channels. The antiinflammatory effects are afforded by inhibition of inflammatory cytokines, including interleukin-1, tumor necrosis factor-alpha, and nuclear factor-kB.[19] A retrospective study examining the survival time of canine subjects with septic peritonitis revealed that subjects receiving lidocaine infusion had improved short-term survival in comparison with those that did not receive it.[2] Lidocaine is a Vaughan Williams Class IB antiarrhythmic agent via blockade of sodium channels in the His-Purkinje system and ventricles, suppressing automaticity and hyperpolarizing cell membranes in this region of the heart.[20] This drug represents the intravenous treatment of choice for ventricular arrhythmias in most species and it has been shown to reduce the minimum alveolar concentration (MAC) of inhalant anesthetics in several species, including dogs[21–24] and cats.[25]

The effect of lidocaine infusion on GI motility is less clear. It has been shown to enhance motility in humans[26] and in horses with postoperative ileus.[27,28] However, it seems to decrease the GI transit time in healthy adult horses.[29] In dogs receiving lidocaine infusion at 50 µg/kg/min, no statistical difference was detected from placebo in regard to GI transit time.[30] Further studies are needed to determine if dogs with compromised GI motility would benefit from lidocaine infusion.

Interestingly, the systemic administration of lidocaine in cats at rates required to reduce MAC causes cardiovascular depression that is more significant compared with the use of inhalant alone at equipotent doses.[25] Furthermore, lidocaine does not reduce the thermal threshold in this species and, therefore, may be less useful for the management of pain.[31]

TOXICITY
Systemic Toxicity

Administration of local anesthetics can cause neurotoxicity and cardiotoxicity as plasma levels increase. Neurotoxicity results from the action of local anesthetics blocking inhibitory pathways within the brain, which leads to unopposed excitatory activity with clinical signs, such as twitching and seizures.[32] As plasma levels continue to increase, cardiotoxic effects will occur due to blockade of sodium channels, resulting in a decrease in the rise of phase 0 of the cardiac action potential.[33] Associated changes on the electrocardiogram (ECG) may be observed, including prolonged PR and QRS intervals.

In general, systemic toxicity is more likely to occur with agents having high lipid solubility (ie, bupivacaine, etidocaine, tetracaine). Additionally, the S-enantiomers are less toxic than the R-enantiomers, making levobupivacaine and ropivacaine safer than their dextrorotary counterparts.[34]

Treatment of local anesthetic systemic toxicity depends on the level of severity. Supportive care should be initiated, including oxygen supplementation and manual ventilation if necessary. If the patient is exhibiting signs of seizure activity, a benzodiazepine should be administered. Careful monitoring of the patient's cardiovascular status should be pursued in order to rule out life-threatening cardiac toxicity. Should cardiovascular depression be encountered, judicious use of fluid support and inotropes may be all that is necessary to restore normal cardiovascular parameters. Cardiac arrhythmias should not be treated with further administration of sodium channel blockers.[35] Alternatively, amiodarone is recommended for the management of ventricular arrhythmias associated with local anesthetic overdose.[35] If cardiac arrest or a malignant ventricular arrhythmia should occur, cardiopulmonary resuscitation should be initiated immediately. Vasopressin and calcium channel blockers should be avoided. Intravenous lipid emulsion has been shown to be effective for treatment of refractory arrhythmias caused by local anesthetic overdose.[36]

Local Toxicity

Neurotoxicity can result from direct injury to the nerve cells when local anesthetics are applied.[37] Chondrotoxicity is a common sequelae of injection of local anesthetics into joint spaces[38]; therefore, intraarticular administration is discouraged. Finally, myotoxicity has also been reported after administration of local anesthetics into skeletal muscle.[39]

Methemoglobinemia

Local anesthetics have the potential to cause oxidative damage to hemoglobin, resulting in the formation of methemoglobin. Benzocaine and prilocaine are the agents most commonly associated with the development of methemoglobinemia.[40]

SPECIAL PREPARATIONS
Lidocaine Patches

Lidocaine patches were introduced in human medicine in the early 1990s and approved in 1999 by the US Food and Drug Administration (FDA) for the treatment of neuropathic pain caused by herpes zoster, commonly known as shingles.[41] Since then, they have been used in humans for chronic low back pain,[42-44] osteoarthritis,[45] painful idiopathic distal sensory polyneuropathy,[46] focal neuropathic pain in patients with cancer,[47] myofascial pain syndrome,[48] and diabetic polyneuropathy.[49] Lidocaine patches have also been used to treat pain after surgical procedures[50-52] and to provide preemptive analgesia.[53]

The lidocaine patch (Lidoderm) is made of a nonwoven polyester felt backing containing adhesive material, and 5% lidocaine (50 mg of lidocaine per gram of adhesive with 700 mg of lidocaine per patch). A release liner protects the adhesive site of the patch and has to be removed before application. The patch is an occlusive delivery system that rehydrates the skin by preventing water loss. The hydration of the stratum corneum enhances the absorption of the drugs through the skin itself.[54] Lidoderm comes in sealed packaging as a nonsterile 10 by 14 cm patch and can be cut to the desired size before application.

In humans, a decrease in pain without numbness or loss of normal sensitivity to temperature and touch of the area where the patch is applied is described.[55] It has been shown that the systemic absorption of lidocaine is minimal, even when an extended dosage regimen is used,[56] suggesting that the analgesic effect is due to the topical absorption.

The exact mechanism of action is unknown. It is likely that the amount of lidocaine that penetrates the skin is sufficient to block only sodium channels of small and damaged nociceptors but not enough to block the A-ß sensory fibers. The blockade of these channels prevents movement of sodium intracellularly, which stabilizes the nerve fiber membranes and stops the action potential responsible for transduction and transmission of nociception.[57]

In veterinary medicine the pharmacokinetics of lidocaine patches have been described in dogs[58-60] and cats.[61] A study in dogs reported lower plasma concentrations when the hair of the lateral side of the thorax was removed by clipping (group A) versus applying a depilatory agent (group B). The mean peak plasma concentrations of lidocaine in group A and B were 62.94 ng/mL reached at 10.67 hours after application and 103.55 ng/mL after 9.27 hours, respectively. Lidocaine plasma levels decreased rapidly after the patch was removed with an elimination half-life of 3.23 and 2.61 hours in group A and B, respectively. The dogs enrolled in this experiment weighed 9.4 to 14.4 kg and the lidocaine patch was applied for 12 hours.[60] The same investigators conducted a second experiment in dogs in which the patch was left on the clipped skin for 60 hours. The mean peak plasma concentrations were 45.18 ng/mL and were achieved after 24 hours.[60] In another study, 2 lidocaine patches were applied for 72 hours in dogs weighing 18 to 23 kg. The mean peak plasma concentrations were similar to the previous study (72.8 ng/mL at 24 hours), remained at steady state between 24 to 48 hours, and decreased between 48 to 60 hours after application.[59] In a more recent study, the investigators compared the pharmacokinetics of a 5% lidocaine patch placed over a skin incision versus intact skin in dogs. Although none of the dogs showed any adverse effects, the area under the plasma lidocaine concentration versus time curve was significantly higher in the incision group compared with the intact skin.[58] In the cat, lidocaine plasma concentrations steadily increase until 12 hours after the patch is applied and the mean peak plasma concentration (106 ng/mL) occurs at 64 hours.[61] In this study the investigators proved that the lidocaine concentrations in the skin under the patch were much higher than the plasma concentrations, confirming that the systemic absorption of the drug is low.[61] Lidocaine plasma concentrations associated with seizures are 8.2 μg/mL in dogs[62] and 19.6 μg/mL in cats,[63] and peak plasma concentrations reached with lidocaine patches are well below these toxic levels in both species.

In veterinary medicine, lidocaine patches have been used to treat postoperative pain for several surgical procedures, such as laparotomies, thoracotomies, hemilaminectomies, stifle surgery, total ear canal ablations, and amputations.[64–66] The patch is applied at the end of the procedure after skin closure. Because the patch is not sterile, it is recommended either to place sterile gauzes over the incision or to cut the patch and apply it around the surgical wound. The lidocaine patch is self-adhesive; however, the protective liner has to be removed and the skin has to be cleaned before application. A surgical film or a bandage can be used to cover and protect the patch and the surgical site. Based on clinical experience and pharmacokinetic data, recommendations on the number of patches per kilogram have been published.[66] Unfortunately, the clinical efficacy of lidocaine patches used for postoperative pain management in dogs is not supported by published data and no clinical studies have been conducted in cats. Two studies in dogs undergoing hemilaminectomies and ovariohysterectomy concluded that the lidocaine patch did not provide additional analgesia compared with the control group.[64,65]

Liposomal Bupivacaine

Exparel is an extended-release formulation of bupivacaine approved in 2011 by the FDA for postsurgical analgesia in humans and sold by Pacira Pharmaceuticals. In this formulation, the bupivacaine is contained in numerous aqueous chambers separated from each other by lipid membranes. The bilayer structure of these membranes consists of phospholipids, triglycerides, and cholesterol. The chambers containing bupivacaine are combined to form microscopic spherical liposomes with a multivesicular, nonconcentric honeycomb-like structure. With time, the vesicles slowly break down, causing the release of bupivacaine and reorganization of the lipid membrane of the liposomes.[67,68]

Two multicentric, double-blind, randomized, placebo-controlled studies were conducted as part of the FDA approval process.[69,70] The investigators showed that liposomal bupivacaine provided extended pain relief superior to placebo up to 48 hours after bunionectomy[69] and 72 hours after hemorrhoidectomy.[70] Both clinical trials reported that the subjects in the treatment group used less opioid postoperatively and adverse effects were considered mild and less frequent than in the placebo group.[69,70]

After the approval, Exparel has been used extensively in human medicine for a variety of soft tissue and orthopedic surgeries. A randomized, double-blind, active-control study compared the efficacy of the liposomal bupivacaine to bupivacaine hydrogen chloride (HCl) mixed with epinephrine for bilateral, cosmetic, submuscular augmentation mammaplasty.[71] Although the study was underpowered, there was a trend of better analgesia and decreased opioid consumption in the prolonged-release bupivacaine group. Another study was conducted in adult subjects undergoing open colectomy.[72] The investigator reported that, when liposomal bupivacaine-based multimodal analgesic regimen was used for postoperative analgesia, opioid consumption, hospitalization time, and costs decreased. Khalil and colleagues[73] compared Exparel administered via intercostal block versus standard continuous thoracic epidural for analgesia after thoracotomies. Subjects receiving the intercostal block reported lower pain scores at day 1 and 3 and had a slightly lower average hospital length of stay.

The efficacy of liposome-encapsulated bupivacaine administered via ultrasound-guided transversus abdominis plane (TAP) block has been evaluated in subjects undergoing abdominal surgery.[74–77] A prospective, single-arm cohort study reported low postsurgical pain scores, high subject satisfaction, and lack of opioid adverse effects when a TAP block was used in subjects undergoing umbilical hernia repair.[74] The limitations of this study included a small number of cases (only 13) and the lack of a control group. Similar results were published by Keller and colleagues[76] in a pilot study and by Stokes and colleagues[77] in a retrospective cohort study. Both groups reported that subjects undergoing colorectal procedures managed with a TAP block using liposomal bupivacaine required less intraoperative and postoperative opioid administration. The treatment group also showed lower pain scores and decreased hospitalization time.[76,77] More recently, a single-institution, parallel-group, open-label randomized trial compared extended-released bupivacaine via TAP block versus continuous epidural injection in subjects undergoing colorectal surgery.[75] The investigators concluded that the use of opioids and cost were greater for the epidural group; however, no differences were found in pain scores, complications, GI recovery, and hospital length of stay. A more recent and comprehensive meta-analysis on the efficacy of liposomal bupivacaine in colorectal resections showed that this drug was associated with decreased opioid use, hospitalization, and pain score. However, hospitalization costs were similar to the control groups.[78]

Most of the human literature on liposomal bupivacaine used for orthopedic procedures is focused on postsurgical analgesia for total knee arthroplasty (TKA).[79–85] The results published for these studies are controversial. A randomized, multicenter, parallel-group, double-blind, dose-ranging study showed that periarticular liposomal bupivacaine provided greater analgesia while subjects were at rest compared with bupivacaine HCl. However, no differences were found in pain during activity, opioid consumption, and resumption to normal daily activity.[80] No difference in pain scores and narcotic use was found in 2 prospective studies in which Exparel was compared with bupivacaine HCl[85] and a modified Ranawat suspension (ropivacaine, epinephrine, ketorolac, and clonidine)[81] administered via periarticular injection. Similar results were published by Pichler and colleagues[84] in a retrospective cohort study. The investigators concluded that liposomal bupivacaine did not decrease inpatient opioid prescriptions and opioid-related complications. Furthermore, Bagsby and colleagues[79] showed that the extended-release bupivacaine provided inferior pain control after 24 hours compared with the traditional and less expensive periarticular injection. These results are in contrast with a more recent phase 4, randomized, double-blind, active-controlled, parallel-group study conducted at 16 centers in the United States.[86] The investigators concluded that patients treated with liposomal bupivacaine had significantly lower pain scores and reduced total opioid consumption. Exparel had been also administered via femoral nerve block for postsurgical analgesia after TKA.[82] The study reported that the treated group had modestly lower pain scores and decreased opioid consumption than the placebo group.

Liposomal bupivacaine seems to have an equal or better safety profile than bupivacaine HCl. The incidence of adverse events is low when recommended doses are administered and the incidence of these side effects is lower when compared with bupivacaine HCl.[87,88] The most common adverse effects are nausea, constipation, and vomiting. Tachycardia and bradycardia have also been reported; however, these were considered mild to moderate in severity and did not require any therapeutic interventions.[88] ECGs and cardiovascular adverse events were evaluated in a phase 2, randomized, double-blind, dose-ranging study of liposomal bupivacaine. In the same report, the investigators analyzed data from 4 phase 1 studies in which either ECG or Holter monitor findings were assessed. The results showed no cardiac adverse effects.[89] When the recommended dose (266 mg total) is used periarticular in TKA, systemic bupivacaine levels remain well below reported cardiac and neurotoxic levels.[90]

In an experimental settings, Ilfeld and colleagues[91] demonstrated that liposomal bupivacaine, bupivacaine HCl, and saline have similar safety profiles when administered via different peripheral nerve blocks. The only side effect observed in rabbits and dogs receiving 9, 18, or either 25 or 30 mg/kg (approximately 1.5, 3, and 5 times the maximum labeled dose of Nocita in dogs; see later discussion) was minimal-to-moderate granulomatous inflammation of the injection site.[92,93] In the first study, the extended-release bupivacaine was administered via infiltration in a inguinal hernia model.[92] In the second study, animals received the study drug via brachial plexus nerve block.[93] The same doses repeated twice weekly for 4 consecutive weeks were administered subcutaneously in a toxicology study in dogs and rabbits.[94] This regimen was well-tolerated in dogs that only showed signs of minimal-to-moderate granulomatous inflammation at the site of injection. In rabbits, convulsions and 1 death were noted.

It seems that when Exparel is administered via intraarticular injection in pigs the chondrocyte viability is preserved.[95] Furthermore, liposomal bupivacaine was well-tolerated in humans when administered via a single epidural injection to heathy volunteers.[96] When the label dose for hemorrhoidectomy (266 mg) was used, motor blockade only lasted 1 hour versus 2.8 hours when compared with 50 mg of bupivacaine HCl. However, pinprick and cold sensitivity loss were 36 and 69 hours, respectively, in the liposomal bupivacaine group versus 12 hours for both in the bupivacaine HCl group.

The equivalent prolonged-release liposomal bupivacaine formulation was introduced in veterinary medicine under the trade name of Nocita and was approved by the FDA in 2016 for postoperative analgesia lasting up to 72 hours for cranial cruciate ligament surgery in dogs. In May 2018, the pharmaceutical company, Aratana Therapeutics, Inc, also obtained the approval for peripheral nerve block for onychectomy in cats.[97] Nocita is a sterile, preservative-free, white to off-white aqueous suspension that comes in 20 mL vials at a concentration of 13.3 mg/mL. The cost of 1 vial (at the time of this publication) ranges from approximately from $170 to $200. According to the manufacturer, unopen vials should be stored in the refrigerator at a temperature between 36°F to 46°F (2°C to 8°C). Alternatively, unopen vials can be stored at room temperature of 68°F to 77°F (20°C to 25°C) for up to 30 days; however, if removed from refrigeration, the drug should never be re-refrigerated. If the drug is exposed to high temperatures (greater than 104°F or 40°C) or is suspected of having been frozen, it should be discarded. Before withdrawing the product into a syringe, the vial should be inverted several times to resuspend the particles but should never be shaken. The vial can then be punctured and the whole content should be withdrawn into syringes (1 per patient) and used within 4 hours. The vial can be punctured only once using aseptic technique.[97]

The label states to avoid concurrent administration of Nocita with bupivacaine HCl or other local anesthetics[97]; however, the Exparel label mentions that the drug may be administered 20 minutes after injection of lidocaine.[98] A review paper on compatibility of liposomal bupivacaine with other drug products and implant materials showed that coadministration of liposomal bupivacaine and bupivacaine HCl at a ratio greater than or equal to 2:1 increased the release of free bupivacaine by only 5% or less.[99] Although the conclusion of the study is that these 2 drugs can be administered together in the same surgical site, the potential additive toxic effects have not been investigated. Other local anesthetics, such as lidocaine, ropivacaine, and mepivacaine, administered together with liposomal bupivacaine tend to displace the drug from the liposomes.[99] When lidocaine was used, this displacement resulted in higher maximum bupivacaine and lidocaine plasma levels in Yucatan miniature pigs compared with plasma levels of animals receiving Exparel and lidocaine alone. However, when an interval of at least 20 minutes was allowed, bupivacaine and lidocaine plasma levels were similar to those of animals receiving the 2 drugs separately.

In the dog, the recommended dose (5.3 mg/kg equal to 0.4 mL/kg) should be infiltrated in the tissues surrounding the surgical site using a moving-needle injection technique.[100] A 25 gauge or larger, 1 to 1.5 inch long needle is inserted up to the hub parallel to the incision. After aspiration to avoid intravascular administration, the drug is delivered as the needle is pulled out. This injection should be repeated by inserting the needle 1 to 1.5 inches from the previous injection site to cover the whole site of the incision. The moving-needle injection technique should be used to infiltrate deep and superficial layers of the surgical site. Before the wound closure, approximately 25%, 50%, and 25% of the total volume should be injected in the tissues around the joint capsule, fascial tissues, and the subcuticular layer, respectively.[101] If the volume is not sufficient, the drug can be diluted up to 1:1 with 0.9% sterile saline or lactated Ringer solution. Data from a pooled analysis of 9 clinical studies showed that this volume expansion does not affect the clinical efficacy or the pharmacokinetics of the drug.[102]

Although several studies have been published on liposomal bupivacaine in dogs,[92–94,101] only 1 investigated the clinical efficacy in this species.[101] In this masked, randomized, placebo-controlled, multicenter pilot field study, dogs undergoing cranial cruciate ligament surgery received liposomal bupivacaine (n = 24) or saline (n = 22) via infiltration of the surgical site before wound closure. The investigators concluded that animals receiving the treatment had significantly lower pain scores versus placebo and that the drug provided measurable local analgesia up to 72 hours after surgery.

In the cat, the approved dose for onychectomy is 5.3 mg/kg per forelimb (0.4 mL/kg per forelimb), for a total dose of 10.6 mg/kg per cat. Four injections should be administered to each forelimb: (1) 0.14 mL/kg (35% of 0.4 mL/kg total) to block the superficial branch of the radial nerve, (2) 0.08 mL/kg (20%) for the dorsal branch of the ulnar nerve, (3) 0.16 mL/kg (40%) for median nerve and superficial branch of the palmar branch of the ulnar nerve, and (4) 0.02 mL/kg (5%) deep branch of the palmar branch of the ulnar nerve.[97]

Currently, no studies have been published on the use of Nocita in cats. As part of the FDA approval process, Aratana Therapeutics conducted 2 studies, 1 on effectiveness and the other to assess the safety profile in cats.[97] The first trial was a masked, randomized, placebo-controlled, multicenter field study conducted in 241 cats undergoing onychectomy. The percentage of cats that needed rescue analgesia within 24, 48, and 72 hours after surgery was 24.8%, 31.3%, and 31.6%, respectively, in the Nocita group and 59.7%, 65.3%, and 64.7%, respectively, in the placebo group. The safety study included 40 healthy cats (4 cats per sex per group) receiving saline at 2.37 mL/kg (negative control) or Nocita at 5.3 mg/kg (active control), 10.6, 21.2, or 31.8 mg/kg (corresponding to 1, 2, and 3 times the maximum labeled dose, respectively). The drug was administered via femoral nerve block on days 0, 9, and 18. One cat in the active control group died during recovery from anesthesia after the second dose for unknown reasons. A cat receiving 31.8 mg/kg was euthanized on day 15 due to a suppurative necrotic wound in the injection site. All the other subjects survived. Clinical side effects in all groups included soft or watery stool and swelling, abrasions, or scabbing around the injection site. Signs of subacute or chronic inflammation around the femoral nerve were noted on the histopathology report.

Liposomal bupivacaine has the potential of becoming 1 of the few options for managing postsurgical pain currently when the availability of opioid drugs is becoming alarmingly limited. Although it has been used experimentally via different block modalities, only local tissue infiltration for cranial cruciate ligament surgery in dogs and peripheral nerve block for onychectomy in cats has been approved. Further clinical trials are needed to assess the efficacy and safety of this formulation administered via different routes and for different surgical procedures in veterinary medicine.

REFERENCES

1. Grzybowski A. Cocaine and the eye: a historical overview. Ophthalmologica 2008;222(5):296–301.

2. Bellini L, Seymour CJ. Effect of intraoperative constant rate infusion of lidocaine on short-term survival of dogs with septic peritonitis: 75 cases (2007-2011). J Am Vet Med Assoc 2016;248(4):422–9.

3. Ruetsch YA, Boni T, Borgeat A. From cocaine to ropivacaine: the history of local anesthetic drugs. Curr Top Med Chem 2001;1(3):175–82.

4. Cousins MJ, Bridenbaugh PO, Carr DB, et al. Cousins and Bridenbaugh's neural blockade in clinical anesthesia and pain medicine 4th ed. Philadelphia: Lippincott Williams & Wilkins; 2009.

5. Narahashi T, Frazier DT. Site of action and active form of local anesthetics. Neurosci Res (N Y) 1971;4:65–99.

6. Butterworth JFT, Strichartz GR. Molecular mechanisms of local anesthesia: a review. Anesthesiology 1990;72(4):711–34.

7. Gissen AJ, Covino BG, Gregus J. Differential sensitivity of fast and slow fibers in mammalian nerve. II. Margin of safety for nerve transmission. Anesth Analg 1982;61(7):561–9.

8. Tucker GT, Boyes RN, Bridenbaugh PO, et al. Binding of anilide-type local anesthetics in human plasma. I. Relationships between binding, physicochemical properties, and anesthetic activity. Anesthesiology 1970;33(3):287–303.

9. Catterall WA. From ionic currents to molecular mechanisms: the structure and function of voltage-gated sodium channels. Neuron 2000;26(1):13–25.

10. Wann KT. Neuronal sodium and potassium channels: structure and function. Br J Anaesth 1993;71(1):2–14.

11. Fozzard HA, Lee PJ, Lipkind GM. Mechanism of local anesthetic drug action on voltage-gated sodium channels. Curr Pharm Des 2005;11(21):2671–86.

12. Hille B. Local anesthetics: hydrophilic and hydrophobic pathways for the drug-receptor reaction. J Gen Physiol 1977;69(4):497–515.

13. Dickey EJ, McKenzie HC 3rd, Brown KA, et al. Serum concentrations of lidocaine and its metabolites after prolonged infusion in healthy horses. Equine Vet J 2008;40(4):348–52.

14. Tobin T, Blake JW, Sturma L, et al. Pharmacology of procaine in the horse: procaine esterase properties of equine plasma and synovial fluid. Am J Vet Res 1976;37(10):1165–70.

15. Cuvillon P, Nouvellon E, Ripart J, et al. A comparison of the pharmacodynamics and pharmacokinetics of bupivacaine, ropivacaine (with epinephrine) and their equal volume mixtures with lidocaine used for femoral and sciatic nerve blocks: a double-blind randomized study. Anesth Analg 2009;108(2):641–9.

16. Galindo A, Witcher T. Mixtures of local anesthetics: bupivacaine-chloroprocaine. Anesth Analg 1980;59(9):683–5.

17. Ribotsky BM, Berkowitz KD, Montague JR. Local anesthetics. Is there an advantage to mixing solutions? J Am Podiatr Med Assoc 1996;86(10):487–91.

18. Sepehripour S, Dheansa BS. Is there an advantage in onset of action with mixing lignocaine and bupivacaine? J Plast Reconstr Aesthet Surg 2017;70(12):1782.

19. Hollmann MW, Durieux ME. Local anesthetics and the inflammatory response: a new therapeutic indication? Anesthesiology 2000;93(3):858–75.

20. Vaughan Williams EM. The relevance of cellular to clinical electrophysiology in classifying antiarrhythmic actions. J Cardiovasc Pharmacol 1992;20(Suppl 2):S1–7.

21. Muir WW 3rd, Wiese AJ, March PA. Effects of morphine, lidocaine, ketamine, and morphine-lidocaine-ketamine drug combination on minimum alveolar concentration in dogs anesthetized with isoflurane. Am J Vet Res 2003;64(9):1155–60.

22. Reed R, Doherty T. Minimum alveolar concentration: key concepts and a review of its pharmacological reduction in dogs. Part 2. Res Vet Sci 2018;118:27–33.

23. Valverde A, Doherty TJ, Hernandez J, et al. Effect of lidocaine on the minimum alveolar concentration of isoflurane in dogs. Vet Anaesth Analg 2004;31(4):264–71.

24. Wilson J, Doherty TJ, Egger CM, et al. Effects of intravenous lidocaine, ketamine, and the combination on the minimum alveolar concentration of sevoflurane in dogs. Vet Anaesth Analg 2008;35(4):289–96.

25. Pypendop BH, Ilkiw JE. The effects of intravenous lidocaine administration on the minimum alveolar concentration of isoflurane in cats. Anesth Analg 2005;100(1):97–101.

26. McCarthy GC, Megalla SA, Habib AS. Impact of intravenous lidocaine infusion on postoperative analgesia and recovery from surgery: a systematic review of randomized controlled trials. Drugs 2010;70(9):1149–63.

27. Brianceau P, Chevalier H, Karas A, et al. Intravenous lidocaine and small-intestinal size, abdominal fluid, and outcome after colic surgery in horses. J Vet Intern Med 2002;16(6):736–41.

28. Malone E, Ensink J, Turner T, et al. Intravenous continuous infusion of lidocaine for treatment of equine ileus. Vet Surg 2006;35(1):60–6.

29. Rusiecki KE, Nieto JE, Puchalski SM, et al. Evaluation of continuous infusion of lidocaine on gastrointestinal tract function in normal horses. Vet Surg 2008;37(6):564–70.

30. Johnson RA, Kierski KR, Jones BG. Evaluation of gastric emptying time, gastrointestinal transit time, sedation score, and nausea score associated with intravenous constant rate infusion of lidocaine hydrochloride in clinically normal dogs. Am J Vet Res 2017;78(5):550–7.

31. Pypendop BH, Ilkiw JE, Robertson SA. Effects of intravenous administration of lidocaine on the thermal threshold in cats. Am J Vet Res 2006;67(1):16–20.
32. Cox B, Durieux ME, Marcus MA. Toxicity of local anaesthetics. Best Pract Res Clin Anaesthesiol 2003;17(1):111–36.
33. Beecroft C, Davies G. Systemic toxic effects of local anaesthetics. Anaesth Intensive Care Med 2013;14(4):146–8.
34. Aberg G. Toxicological and local anaesthetic effects of optically active isomers of two local anaesthetic compounds. Acta Pharmacol Toxicol (Copenh) 1972; 31(4):273–86.
35. Weinberg GL. Current concepts in resuscitation of patients with local anesthetic cardiac toxicity. Reg Anesth Pain Med 2002;27(6):568–75.
36. Weinberg G, Ripper R, Feinstein DL, et al. Lipid emulsion infusion rescues dogs from bupivacaine-induced cardiac toxicity. Reg Anesth Pain Med 2003;28(3): 198–202.
37. Verlinde M, Hollmann MW, Stevens MF, et al. Local anesthetic-induced neuro-toxicity. Int J Mol Sci 2016;17(3):339.
38. Baker JF, Mulhall KJ. Local anaesthetics and chondrotoxicty: what is the evidence? Knee Surg Sports Traumatol Arthrosc 2012;20(11):2294–301.
39. Hussain N, McCartney CJL, Neal JM, et al. Local anaesthetic-induced myotoxicity in regional anaesthesia: a systematic review and empirical analysis. Br J Anaesth 2018;121(4):822–41.
40. Davis JA, Greenfield RE, Brewer TG. Benzocaine-induced methemoglobinemia attributed to topical application of the anesthetic in several laboratory animal species. Am J Vet Res 1993;54(8):1322–6.
41. Rowbotham MC, Davies PS, Verkempinck C, et al. Lidocaine patch: double-blind controlled study of a new treatment method for post-herpetic neuralgia. Pain 1996;65(1):39–44.
42. Galer BS, Gammaitoni AR, Oleka N, et al. Use of the lidocaine patch 5% in reducing intensity of various pain qualities reported by patients with low-back pain. Curr Med Res Opin 2004;20(Suppl 2):S5–12.
43. Gimbel J, Linn R, Hale M, et al. Lidocaine patch treatment in patients with low back pain: results of an open-label, nonrandomized pilot study. Am J Ther 2005;12(4):311–9.
44. Hines R, Keaney D, Moskowitz MH, et al. Use of lidocaine patch 5% for chronic low back pain: a report of four cases. Pain Med 2002;3(4):361–5.
45. Gammaitoni AR, Galer BS, Onawola R, et al. Lidocaine patch 5% and its positive impact on pain qualities in osteoarthritis: results of a pilot 2-week, open-label study using the Neuropathic Pain Scale. Curr Med Res Opin 2004;20(Suppl 2):S13–9.
46. Herrmann DN, Barbano RL, Hart-Gouleau S, et al. An open-label study of the lidocaine patch 5% in painful idiopathic sensory polyneuropathy. Pain Med 2005;6(5):379–84.
47. Lopez Ramirez E. Treatment of acute and chronic focal neuropathic pain in cancer patients with lidocaine 5 % patches. A radiation and oncology department experience. Support Care Cancer 2013;21(5):1329–34.
48. Lin YC, Kuan TS, Hsieh PC, et al. Therapeutic effects of lidocaine patch on myofascial pain syndrome of the upper trapezius: a randomized, double-blind, placebo-controlled study. Am J Phys Med Rehabil 2012;91(10):871–82.
49. Barbano RL, Herrmann DN, Hart-Gouleau S, et al. Effectiveness, tolerability, and impact on quality of life of the 5% lidocaine patch in diabetic polyneuropathy. Arch Neurol 2004;61(6):914–8.

50. Gilhooly D, McGarvey B, O'Mahony H, et al. Topical lidocaine patch 5% for acute postoperative pain control. BMJ Case Rep 2011;2011 [pii:bcr0620103074].

51. Habib AS, Polascik TJ, Weizer AZ, et al. Lidocaine patch for postoperative analgesia after radical retropubic prostatectomy. Anesth Analg 2009;108(6):1950–3.

52. Saber AA, Elgamal MH, Rao AJ, et al. Early experience with lidocaine patch for postoperative pain control after laparoscopic ventral hernia repair. Int J Surg 2009;7(1):36–8.

53. Kim KH. Use of lidocaine patch for percutaneous endoscopic lumbar discectomy. Korean J Pain 2011;24(2):74–80.

54. Riviere JE, Papich MG. Potential and problems of developing transdermal patches for veterinary applications. Adv Drug Deliv Rev 2001;50(3):175–203.

55. Pasero C. Pain control: lidocaine patch 5%. Am J Nurs 2003;103:75–8.

56. Gammaitoni AR, Davis MW. Pharmacokinetics and tolerability of lidocaine patch 5% with extended dosing. Ann Pharmacother 2002;36(2):236–40.

57. Gammaitoni AR, Alvarez NA, Galer BS. Safety and tolerability of the lidocaine patch 5%, a targeted peripheral analgesic: a review of the literature. J Clin Pharmacol 2003;43(2):111–7.

58. Joudrey SD, Robinson DA, Kearney MT, et al. Plasma concentrations of lidocaine in dogs following lidocaine patch application over an incision compared to intact skin. J Vet Pharmacol Ther 2015;38(6):575–80.

59. Ko J, Weil A, Maxwell L, et al. Plasma concentrations of lidocaine in dogs following lidocaine patch application. J Am Anim Hosp Assoc 2007;43(5):280–3.

60. Weiland L, Croubels S, Baert K, et al. Pharmacokinetics of a lidocaine patch 5% in dogs. J Vet Med A Physiol Pathol Clin Med 2006;53(1):34–9.

61. Ko JC, Maxwell LK, Abbo LA, et al. Pharmacokinetics of lidocaine following the application of 5% lidocaine patches to cats. J Vet Pharmacol Ther 2008;31(4):359–67.

62. Wilcke JR, Davis LE, Neff-Davis CA. Determination of lidocaine concentrations producing therapeutic and toxic effects in dogs. J Vet Pharmacol Ther 1983;6(2):105–11.

63. de Jong RH, Ronfeld RA, DeRosa RA. Cardiovascular effects of convulsant and supraconvulsant doses of amide local anesthetics. Anesth Analg 1982;61(1):3–9.

64. Merema DK, Schoenrock EK, Le Boedec K, et al. Effects of a transdermal lidocaine patch on indicators of postoperative pain in dogs undergoing midline ovariohysterectomy. J Am Vet Med Assoc 2017;250(10):1140–7.

65. Re Bravo V, Aprea F, Bhalla RJ, et al. Effect of 5% transdermal lidocaine patches on postoperative analgesia in dogs undergoing hemilaminectomy. J Small Anim Pract 2018;60(3):161–6.

66. Weil AB, Ko J, Inoue T. The use of lidocaine patches. Compend Contin Educ Vet 2007;29(4):208–10, 212, 214-206.

67. Lascelles BDX, Kirkby Shaw K. An extended release local anaesthetic: potential for future use in veterinary surgical patients? Vet Med Sci 2016;2(4):229–38.

68. Simone A. Center for drug evaluation and research, clinical review NDA 022-496 Exparel (bupivacaine). Food and Drug Administration (FDA). 2011. Availble at: https://www.accessdata.fda.gov/drugsatfda_docs/nda/2011/022496Orig1s000 MedR.pdf. Accessed January 10, 2019.

69. Golf M, Daniels SE, Onel E. A phase 3, randomized, placebo-controlled trial of DepoFoam® bupivacaine (extended-release bupivacaine local analgesic) in bunionectomy. Adv Ther 2011;28(9):776–88.

70. Gorfine SR, Onel E, Patou G, et al. Bupivacaine extended-release liposome injection for prolonged postsurgical analgesia in patients undergoing hemorrhoidectomy: a multicenter, randomized, double-blind, placebo-controlled trial. Dis Colon Rectum 2011;54(12):1552–9.

71. Smoot JD, Bergese SD, Onel E, et al. The efficacy and safety of DepoFoam bupivacaine in patients undergoing bilateral, cosmetic, submuscular augmentation mammaplasty: a randomized, double-blind, active-control study. Aesthet Surg J 2012;32(1):69–76.

72. Cohen SM. Extended pain relief trial utilizing infiltration of Exparel(®), a long-acting multivesicular liposome formulation of bupivacaine: a Phase IV health economic trial in adult patients undergoing open colectomy. J Pain Res 2012; 5:567–72.

73. Khalil KG, Boutrous ML, Irani AD, et al. Operative intercostal nerve blocks with long-acting bupivacaine liposome for pain control after thoracotomy. Ann Thorac Surg 2015;100(6):2013–8.

74. Feierman DE, Kronenfeld M, Gupta PM, et al. Liposomal bupivacaine infiltration into the transversus abdominis plane for postsurgical analgesia in open abdominal umbilical hernia repair: results from a cohort of 13 patients. J Pain Res 2014; 7:477–82.

75. Felling DR, Jackson MW, Ferraro J, et al. Liposomal bupivacaine transversus abdominis plane block versus epidural analgesia in a colon and rectal surgery enhanced recovery pathway: a randomized clinical trial. Dis Colon Rectum 2018;61(10):1196–204.

76. Keller DS, Tahilramani RN, Flores-Gonzalez JR, et al. Pilot study of a novel pain management strategy: evaluating the impact on patient outcomes. Surg Endosc 2016;30(6):2192–8.

77. Stokes AL, Adhikary SD, Quintili A, et al. Liposomal bupivacaine use in transversus abdominis plane blocks reduces pain and postoperative intravenous opioid requirement after colorectal surgery. Dis Colon Rectum 2017;60(2):170–7.

78. Raman S, Lin M, Krishnan N. Systematic review and meta-analysis of the efficacy of liposomal bupivacaine in colorectal resections. J Drug Assess 2018; 7(1):43–50.

79. Bagsby DT, Ireland PH, Meneghini RM. Liposomal bupivacaine versus traditional periarticular injection for pain control after total knee arthroplasty. J Arthroplasty 2014;29(8):1687–90.

80. Bramlett K, Onel E, Viscusi ER, et al. A randomized, double-blind, dose-ranging study comparing wound infiltration of DepoFoam bupivacaine, an extended-release liposomal bupivacaine, to bupivacaine HCl for postsurgical analgesia in total knee arthroplasty. Knee 2012;19(5):530–6.

81. Collis PN, Hunter AM, Vaughn MD, et al. Periarticular injection after total knee arthroplasty using liposomal bupivacaine vs a modified ranawat suspension: a prospective, randomized study. J Arthroplasty 2016;31(3):633–6.

82. Hadzic A, Minkowitz HS, Melson TI, et al. Liposome bupivacaine femoral nerve block for postsurgical analgesia after total knee arthroplasty. Anesthesiology 2016;124(6):1372–83.

83. Hyland SJ, Deliberato DG, Fada RA, et al. Liposomal bupivacaine versus standard periarticular injection in total knee arthroplasty with regional anesthesia: a prospective randomized controlled trial. J Arthroplasty 2019;34(3): 488–94.

84. Pichler L, Poeran J, Zubizarreta N, et al. Liposomal bupivacaine does not reduce inpatient opioid prescription or related complications after knee arthroplasty: a database analysis. Anesthesiology 2018;129(4):689–99.

85. Schroer WC, Diesfeld PG, LeMarr AR, et al. Does extended-release liposomal bupivacaine better control pain than bupivacaine after total knee arthroplasty (TKA)? A prospective, randomized clinical trial. J Arthroplasty 2015;30(9 Suppl):64–7.

86. Mont MA, Beaver WB, Dysart SH, et al. Local infiltration analgesia with liposomal bupivacaine improves pain scores and reduces opioid use after total knee arthroplasty: results of a randomized controlled trial. J Arthroplasty 2018; 33(1):90–6.

87. Portillo J, Kamar N, Melibary S, et al. Safety of liposome extended-release bupivacaine for postoperative pain control. Front Pharmacol 2014;5:90.

88. Viscusi ER, Sinatra R, Onel E, et al. The safety of liposome bupivacaine, a novel local analgesic formulation. Clin J Pain 2014;30(2):102–10.

89. Bergese SD, Onel E, Morren M, et al. Bupivacaine extended-release liposome injection exhibits a favorable cardiac safety profile. Reg Anesth Pain Med 2012;37(2):145–51.

90. Springer BD, Mason JB, Odum SM. Systemic safety of liposomal bupivacaine in simultaneous bilateral total knee arthroplasty. J Arthroplasty 2018;33(1): 97–101.

91. Ilfeld BM, Viscusi ER, Hadzic A, et al. Safety and side effect profile of liposome bupivacaine (Exparel) in peripheral nerve blocks. Reg Anesth Pain Med 2015; 40(5):572–82.

92. Richard BM, Ott LR, Haan D, et al. The safety and tolerability evaluation of DepoFoam bupivacaine (bupivacaine extended-release liposome injection) administered by incision wound infiltration in rabbits and dogs. Expert Opin Investig Drugs 2011;20(10):1327–41.

93. Richard BM, Newton P, Ott LR, et al. The safety of exparel ® (bupivacaine liposome injectable suspension) administered by peripheral nerve block in rabbits and dogs. J Drug Deliv 2012;2012:962101.

94. Richard BM, Rickert DE, Newton PE, et al. Safety evaluation of Exparel (DepoFoam bupivacaine) administered by repeated subcutaneous injection in rabbits and dogs: species comparison. J Drug Deliv 2011;2011:467429.

95. Shaw KA, Moreland C, Jacobs J, et al. Improved chondrotoxic profile of liposomal bupivacaine compared with standard bupivacaine after intra-articular infiltration in a porcine model. Am J Sports Med 2018;46(1): 66–71.

96. Viscusi ER, Candiotti KA, Onel E, et al. The pharmacokinetics and pharmacodynamics of liposome bupivacaine administered via a single epidural injection to healthy volunteers. Reg Anesth Pain Med 2012;37(6):616–22.

97. Nocita (bupivacaine liposome injectable suspension) [package insert]. Leawood (KS): Aratana Therapeutics, Inc; 2018.

98. Exparel (bupivacaine liposome injectable suspension) [package insert]. San Diego (CA): Pacira Pharmaceuticals, Inc; 2014.

99. Kharitonov V. A review of the compatibility of liposome bupivacaine with other drug products and commonly used implant materials. Postgrad Med 2014; 126(1):129–38.

100. Aratana therapeutics. Dosing and administration. 2019. Available at: https://nocita.aratana.com/dosingandadministration-2. Accessed February 10, 2019.

101. Lascelles BD, Rausch-Derra LC, Wofford JA, et al. Pilot, randomized, placebo-controlled clinical field study to evaluate the effectiveness of bupivacaine liposome injectable suspension for the provision of post-surgical analgesia in dogs undergoing stifle surgery. BMC Vet Res 2016;12(1):168.
102. Hadzic A, Abikhaled JA, Harmon WJ. Impact of volume expansion on the efficacy and pharmacokinetics of liposome bupivacaine. Local Reg Anesth 2015; 8:105–11.

Adjuvant Analgesics in Acute Pain Management

Hélène L.M. Ruel, DMV, MSc, Paulo V. Steagall, MV, MSc, PhD*

KEYWORDS

- Gabapentin • Ketamine • Tramadol • Canine • Feline • Adjuvant drugs • Analgesia
- Pain

KEY POINTS

- The efficacy of gabapentin in combination with buprenorphine has been demonstrated after ovariohysterectomy in cats. Additional studies using gabapentin alone are required to evaluate its efficacy in dogs and cats.
- The use of ketamine in clinical practice, including dosage regimens, drug combinations, advantages, disadvantages or limitations, anesthetic-sparing effects, and clinically relevant studies, is presented.
- The analgesic efficacy of tramadol relies on the activity of cytochrome P 450 enzymes to produce its active metabolites (ie, O-desmethyltramadol). Dogs produce less concentrations of this metabolite and tramadol's efficacy has been questioned in this species.
- The use of tramadol in dogs should be judicious. Veterinarians should know the potential for analgesic failure and the clinical limitations of the drug in pain management.

GABAPENTIN
Mechanism of Action and Pharmacology

Gabapentin is a structural analogue of the inhibitory neurotransmitter gamma-aminobutyric acid (GABA); however, it has little activity at the GABA receptors. Instead, it is thought that gabapentinoids exert their main effects by binding to the $\alpha2$-δ subunit of the voltage-gated calcium channels.[1] Gabapentin also inhibits presynaptic release of GABA and induces glutamate release in the locus coeruleus located in the brainstem.[2] Therefore, gabapentin acts also on the descending noradrenergic inhibitory system.[3]

Gabapentin has high oral bioavailability in dogs (80%; 50 mg/kg)[4] and cats (90%–95%; 10 mg/kg).[5,6] Peak plasma concentrations are expected to occur 45 minutes to 2 hours after oral administration in both cats[5,6] and dogs.[7] In dogs, 34% of the drug is metabolized by the liver into N-methyl-gabapentin and it is eliminated by renal

Disclosure Statement: The authors have nothing to disclose.
Department of Clinical Sciences, Faculty of Veterinary Medicine, Université de Montréal, 3200 rue Sicotte, Saint-Hyacinthe, Quebec J2S 2M2, Canada
* Corresponding author.
E-mail address: paulo.steagall@umontreal.ca

excretion.[4] The extensiveness of hepatic biotransformation in cats is unknown. Elimination half-lives are approximately between 3 and 4 hours in dogs and cats.[5,6,8] This information suggests the need for frequent oral dosing. However, specific target-levels for antiepileptic efficacy and pain management are yet to be determined in companion animals.

Some drug interactions have been described in humans but it is unknown if similar effects occur in animals. In humans, coadministration of hydrocodone or morphine may lead to increases in the plasma concentrations of gabapentin. A delay of 2 hours is also recommended when gabapentin is administered concomitantly with aluminum-magnesium hydroxides because they can decrease the absorption of gabapentin.

Clinical Use

Gabapentin is approved by the US Food and Drug Administration as an adjunct anti-epileptic and antihyperalgesic drug (for neuropathic pain associated with postherpetic neuralgia) in humans. The drug is inexpensive and easily available for oral administration in capsules, tablets, or liquid. Some formulations contain xylitol, which can be toxic at large doses in dogs. For this reason, care must be taken when prescribing this drug from a nonveterinary pharmacy. It is currently nonscheduled in most of the United States.

In dogs and cats, gabapentin was initially used off-label as an antiepileptic drug. Despite the limited number of randomized controlled trials and dosage recommendations, the drug is now widely used for chronic pain management. More recently, its analgesic properties for acute and postoperative pain have been investigated in companion animals in combination with other analgesic drugs,[9–12] or administered alone as a single dose to facilitate transportation and examination, or to attenuate fear responses in cage-trap cats.[13,14]

Evidence in Humans Related to Acute Pain

A recent meta-analysis showed that a single dose of gabapentin or pregabalin administered preoperatively reduced opioid consumption in the postoperative period.[15] Gabapentin provided adequate pain control in the early period after cesarean section without increasing maternal or neonatal adverse effects.[16] It also provided superior analgesia when compared with placebo, and it decreased the prevalence of vomiting after craniotomy[17] and open hysterectomy.[18] However, it did not improve pain scores or reduce opioid requirements when used in critically ill patients with rib fractures[19] or before hysterectomy by laparoscopy.[20] A systematic review and meta-analysis is currently being conducted to document the efficacy and safety of gabapentinoids (ie, gabapentin and pregabalin) in the perioperative period to support recommendations of the American Pain Society on the use of perioperative gabapentinoids[21] (**Box 1**).

Evidence in Companion Animals

The World Small Animal Veterinary Association Global Pain Council recommends the perioperative use of gabapentin as an adjunctive treatment to prevent or treat postsurgical pain, or in circumstances of limited availability of analgesic drugs.[23] However, the current knowledge on the analgesic effects of gabapentin in companion animals is mostly based on expert opinion, case reports, and review articles (see **Box 1**).[23–27] For example, the analgesic efficacy of gabapentin has been reported in case series following major orthopedic procedures,[27] wound debridement,[26] musculoskeletal pain, and head trauma.[28] The administration of buprenorphine in combination with 2 preoperative doses of gabapentin (50 mg per cat; 12 hours and 1 hour before

---

Box 1
Current recommendations of the American Society of Pain regarding the use of gabapentin for the management of postoperative pain in humans[22]

- Type of patients
  ○ Patients undergoing major or minor surgery

- Dose range
  ○ For preoperative use: 600 to 1200 mg per individual, to be administered 1 to 2 hours before surgery as part of multimodal analgesia; preoperative use is recommended for major surgery or when high degree of pain is expected.
  ○ For postoperative use: 600 mg per individual as a single or in multiple doses.

- Adverse effects
  ○ Dizziness, fatigue, and sedation without evidence of respiratory depression.
  ○ The dose should be reduced in patients with renal dysfunction.

---

surgery) provided similar analgesic effects to buprenorphine-meloxicam in cats undergoing ovariohysterectomy. Depending on the pain scoring system, buprenorphine-gabapentin provided better pain relief than buprenorphine alone.[11] On the other hand, thermal antinociception and decreases in the minimum alveolar concentration (MAC) of isoflurane were not observed in healthy cats treated with gabapentin.[29,30]

Data on the efficacy of gabapentin alone are lacking in dogs. Perioperative administration of gabapentin (10 mg/kg orally) in combination with intramuscular morphine reduced postoperative morphine consumption following mastectomy when compared with placebo.[10] However, pain scores in dogs undergoing hemilaminectomy or limb amputation, and treated with gabapentin in combination with other analgesics, did not differ from those treated with placebo and other analgesics.[9,12] The concomitant administration of other analgesics is a confounding factor in these studies. In a study performed in the authors' laboratory, dogs with naturally occurring neuropathic pain had lower pain scores when treated medically with gabapentin alone (10 mg/kg orally every 8 hours for 7 days) or in combination with meloxicam (0.2 mg/kg followed by 0.1 mg/kg/d) than baseline (Ruel & Steagall 2019, unpublished observations) (**Box 2**).

Box 2
The most important features of gabapentin for acute pain management in companion animals

- Gabapentin should be administered every 6 to 8 hours orally to sustain plasma concentrations of the drug. Studies using 12-hour intervals of administration showed that gabapentin had poor response.[9,12]

- The plasma concentrations of gabapentin associated with acute pain relief are unknown in companion animals. Based on the human literature and a study in cats,[11] single or double preoperative doses of 15 to 30 mg/kg orally are recommended for postoperative pain relief to reduce opioid consumption. These doses are similar to those used to facilitate transportation and veterinary examination and reduce fear responses in cage-trap cats.[13,14]

- The following doses for chronic pain or persistent postsurgical pain have been suggested:
  ○ Dogs: 10 mg/kg every 8 hours orally[25]
  ○ Cats: 8 mg/kg every 6 hours orally.[5]

- Adverse effects may include sedation and dizziness in humans and are usually self-limited. In companion animals, sedation and ataxia can occur. Loose stools have been reported; however, the association with the administration of gabapentin was not clearly established.[7] Gabapentin seems safe for companion animals.

KETAMINE
Mechanism of Action and Pharmacology

The analgesic effects of ketamine are mostly due to its noncompetitive and nonspecific antagonism of the N-methyl D-aspartate (NMDA) receptors.[31] These receptors are activated by 2 excitatory neurotransmitters (ie, glycine and glutamate) during sustained nociception in the dorsal horn of the spinal cord and are important in the transmission and modulation of nociceptive stimuli (ie, pain facilitation). For this reason, NMDA receptors are key players in central sensitization and cumulative depolarization (so-called wind-up).[32] The activation of NMDA receptors occurs mostly in maladaptive and not in nociceptive pain.[33] Subanesthetic doses of ketamine can antagonize NMDA receptors and produce antihyperalgesic effects; ketamine is not considered a classic stand-alone analgesic. Ketamine also has effects on μ-opioid, muscarinic, monoaminergic, and GABA receptors, among others, which are responsible for some of the systemic effects.[34]

Ketamine at anesthetic doses may suppress natural killer cell activity, which has been shown to promote lung and liver metastases in animal models.[35–37] On the other hand, low-dose ketamine presents some immunomodulatory effects. The drug can reverse pain-induced immunosuppression[38,39] and can suppress proinflammatory cytokine productions (tumor necrosis factor-α and interleukins 6 and 8).[40]

Clinical Use

There has been increasing interest concerning the use of ketamine, especially considering its inhalant and opioid-sparing effects, the current opioid-related public health crisis, and its wide-spread availability. Furthermore, optimal pain relief is often difficult to achieve without significant adverse effects when using a single analgesic, thus multimodal analgesia with ketamine has been recommended in cats with major injury.[26,41]

Subanesthetic doses of ketamine are used as a variable or constant rate infusion (CRI) for pain management in the perioperative period. The administration of single boluses alone for perioperative analgesia is uncommon due to its rapid clearance. Ketamine is mostly administered intravenously in small animal practice, and pain assessment and monitoring is required during the hospitalization. The drug is administered to prevent or treat the hyperalgesia and allodynia commonly associated with central sensitization during major surgery. After surgery, dogs and cats are often transferred to an intermediate or intensive care unit where the infusion is continued for 24 to 72 hours postoperatively.

The activation of NMDA receptors in the central nervous system following traumatic brain injury is associated with poor prognosis. Subanesthetic doses of ketamine are administered for neuroprotection against ischemic brain injury and glutamate-induced brain injury. These low doses (2–16 μ/kg/min) are not associated with increases in intracranial pressure. However, ketamine should be used with caution in these patients when ventilation is already compromised because hypoventilation (ie, increases in $Paco_2$) may lead to increases in intracranial pressure. Anesthetic doses of ketamine are rarely used in patients with increased intracranial pressure because indirect sympathetic activation could increase blood pressure, cerebral blood flow, and cerebral perfusion pressure.

In both dogs and cats, ketamine is excreted by the kidneys, and patients with renal impairment may experience prolonged effect of the drug, especially cats. However, anecdotally, subanesthetic doses of ketamine infusions have been used for postoperative pain control in cats after subcutaneous urethral bypass when renal function is improving over time.

Dosage regimens usually consist of administering a loading dose (0.15–0.7 mg/kg) followed by a CRI (2–10 μg/kg/min) (**Box 3**).[42,43] Ketamine is used in combination with opioids and other analgesics (ie, systemic lidocaine and local anesthetic blocks) but rarely as a first-line analgesic for treatment of pain. Indeed, in a study, ketamine infusions did not provide adequate analgesia in combination with butorphanol; 37.5% of dogs required rescue analgesia after ovariohysterectomy.[44] Pain scores in that study were higher in the ketamine group when compared with dexmedetomidine infusions, or a combination of lidocaine-ketamine-dexmedetomidine (LKD) infusions.

Ketamine may also be combined with opioids to optimize inhalant-sparing effects and improve the quality of anesthesia. This has been the objective of several studies in veterinary anesthesia but one should bear in mind that higher than subanesthetic doses have been used.[45–47] The summary of the clinical use of ketamine is presented in **Box 4**.

Evidence in Humans Related to Acute Pain

Consensus guidelines on the use of intravenous ketamine infusion for acute pain management from the American Society of Regional Anesthesia and Pain Medicine, the American Academy of Pain Medicine, and the American Society of Anesthesiologists have been recently published.[48] Recommendations of the consensus are summarized in **Box 5**. Readers should be aware that recommendations have different grades and suggestions from practice, and have low, moderate, or high levels of certainty (**Box 5**).

Evidence in Veterinary Medicine

Ketamine has shown to improve postoperative analgesia in dogs undergoing forelimb amputation.[43] A ketamine CRI has also been used as an adjunctive analgesic drug in cats undergoing major surgery to minimize the risk of central sensitization and to decrease opioid requirements in the intensive care unit.[26] Adverse effects have not been reported but evidence is low owing to the clinical nature and lack of opioid-based control groups in these studies. In these studies, ketamine was administered in combination with other analgesic techniques, thus it is difficult to appreciate the true analgesic benefits of ketamine for pain relief in this context. Ketamine improved feeding behavior when administered during the postoperative period using a bolus of 0.7 mg/kg followed by a CRI of 10 μg/kg/min in dogs after mastectomy.[42] However, it did not provide an opioid-sparing effect nor induce better analgesia than a control group receiving morphine intravenously in that study. A loading dose followed by a CRI of ketamine in combination with other analgesics has been associated with analgesia of longer duration in dogs undergoing ovariohysterectomy and major surgery.[43,49]

Studies with the use of ketamine for balanced anesthesia have been published especially in terms of dose-dependent decreases in the MAC of inhalant anesthetics,

---

Box 3
A practical approach to ketamine infusion in clinical practice.

- 60 mg of ketamine (0.6 mL of ketamine 10%) can be mixed in 0.5 L of a crystalloid solution. The patient will receive an infusion of 10 μg/kg/min if the infusion is administered at 5 mL/kg/h in the intraoperative period.

- Concentrations and doses should be adjusted in the perioperative period according to fluid therapy rates.

Box 4
The most important features of ketamine and its clinical use

- Ketamine is an NMDA antagonist used for the prevention and treatment of maladaptive pain.
- Dosage regimens usually consist of administering a loading dose (0.15–0.7 mg/kg), followed by variable infusion rates (2–10 μg/kg/min).
- Ketamine is often administered in the perioperative period by the intravenous route, and in combination with opioids, local anesthetic blocks, and nonsteroidal antiinflammatory drugs (ie, multimodal analgesia).

---

in addition to its antihyperalgesic effects.[45–47,50–53] For example, in the absence of a loading dose, a 10 μg/kg/min CRI reduced the MAC of isoflurane by 25%.[51] End-tidal concentrations of isoflurane were reduced up to 28.9% in dogs undergoing ovariohysterectomy when a loading dose of 1 mg/kg followed by 40 μg/kg/min was administered.[46] Finally, a loading dose of 2 mg/kg followed by a CRI of ketamine (1.38 mg/kg/h or 23 μg/kg/min) reduced the mean MAC of isoflurane by 45% in cats.[52] Therefore, doses of ketamine for inhalant anesthetic-sparing are often higher than those previously reported for analgesia.

A combination of remifentanil and ketamine (bolus of 0.5 mg/kg followed by 30 μg/kg/min) infusions provided clinically relevant greater isoflurane-sparing effect when compared with a control group or remifentanil alone after ovariohysterectomy in cats.[54] This effect may be important in ill cats that do not tolerate the cardiorespiratory depression produced by inhalant anesthetics. Analgesic effects were not evaluated in the latter study.

The combination LKD has been investigated in dogs (**Box 6**).[44,46] Isoflurane requirements were significantly reduced during LKD CRI by approximately 55% when compared with controls, ketamine, dexmedetomidine, or lidocaine CRI alone.

Box 5
Summary of recommendations on the use of intravenous ketamine infusion for acute pain management in humans with potential impact in companion animals

- Type of patients
  - Patients undergoing surgery for which postoperative pain will be severe (ie, abdominal, thoracic surgery, and limb and spine procedures)
  - Patients with opioid tolerance or dependence, especially with acute on chronic, acute exacerbation of chronic conditions
  - As an adjuvant to opioid analgesics in perioperative analgesia

- Dose range
  - Common subanesthetic doses vary between 0.3 and 0.5 mg/kg bolus with or without an infusion (0.1–0.2 mg/kg/h or approximately 2–4 μg/kg/min). However, some studies administered up to 80 μg/kg/min.
  - The overall recommendation is not to exceed a bolus of 0.35 mg/kg and an infusion rate of 16 μg/kg/min, with some exceptions.

- Contraindications
  - The human literature does not provide clear guidance on contraindications for ketamine. Therefore, contraindications are often based on the anesthetic use of ketamine (ie, high doses) in patients with uncontrolled cardiovascular disease, pregnancy, and hepatic dysfunction.
  - Contraindications for low-dose ketamine are poorly reported.

Box 6
The use of lidocaine-ketamine-dexmedetomidine in dogs

- A loading dose (2 mg/kg) of lidocaine followed by a CRI of 100 µg/kg/min, a loading dose (1 mg/kg) of ketamine followed by a CRI of 40 µg/kg/min, and a loading dose (1 µg/kg) of dexmedetomidine followed by a CRI of 3 µg/kg/h is used.

- Boluses should be administered slowly (eg, over 60 seconds). They could be either administered before or after induction of anesthesia. The administration before induction of anesthesia may reduce the requirements of injectable anesthetics.

- Volatile anesthetic concentrations should be reduced on a case-by-case basis. Veterinarians should expect a sparing effect of 50% to 60% but could be much more profound in dogs that are sensitive to α_2-adrenoreceptor agonists or in critical condition.

- The technique has not been studied in cats, and these patients may react differently to this drug combination. For this reason, the authors do not recommend this technique in cats until further studies are performed.

However, LKD prolonged anesthetic recovery (time to extubation, time to first head lift, time to sternal recumbency, and time to standing). In the clinical setting, prolonged anesthetic recoveries after LKD CRI could be prevented with the administration of an α_2-adrenoreceptor antagonist (eg, atipamezole) to reverse the sedative and cardiovascular effects of dexmedetomidine but it would also end any analgesic effect associated with this drug. A CRI of LKD was associated with lower pain scores when compared with each drug CRI alone. None of the dogs required rescue analgesia after ovariohysterectomy, and treatment with LKD provided similar analgesia when compared with fentanyl CRI. The LKD protocol is an excellent alternative to opioids for balanced anesthesia in dogs. However, this protocol has not been evaluated in cats and should be used with caution especially considering the deleterious cardiovascular effects of lidocaine in this species.

Anesthetic recoveries after prolonged ketamine infusion rates (ie, 12 hours in MAC studies) have been reported to be rough and protracted in cats.[52] However, other studies have not corroborated these findings, and it seems that subanesthetic doses of ketamine do not impair anesthetic recovery in cats in a short-term basis.[54] Nevertheless, acepromazine can be administered in normovolemic cats to prevent ketamine-induced dysphoria in the early postoperative period.[54]

TRAMADOL
Mechanism of Action

Tramadol is a dual-action analgesic drug. It is a centrally acting synthetic weak opioid agonist and a serotonin and norepinephrine reuptake inhibitor. Therefore, in addition to its opioid effects, tramadol produces central modulation of nociception by enhancing noradrenergic and serotoninergic activity.[55]

Tramadol is metabolized by cytochrome P (CYP)-450 enzymes into active metabolites. The (+)-M1 metabolites bind to the µ-opioid receptor to produce analgesia and are involved in opioid-induced adverse effects. The (+)-O-desmethyltramadol is the most important M1 metabolite. Additionally, the (+)-M5 metabolite (N,O-desmethyltramadol) also contributes to the analgesic effects in some species but its clinical relevance is unknown in companion animals. There are major species differences in the metabolism of tramadol regarding the CYP450 genes and subfamilies (**Box 7**).

The data presented previously suggest that the analgesic efficacy and adverse effects produced by tramadol vary according to the species but also the intrinsic hepatic

---

Box 7
Species-specific differences in the metabolism of tramadol

- Tramadol is catalyzed by CYP2D6 and CYP3A4 in humans, whereas the CYP2D15 is responsible for the production of (+)-M1 metabolites in dogs.

- Both (+)-M1 and (+)-M2 metabolites are transformed into (+)-M5 metabolite in dogs, which is the major by-product of tramadol found in plasma and urine in this species. The complex metabolism of tramadol in dogs has been recently described.[56]

- Oral, epidural, and parenteral administration of tramadol does not lead to significant concentrations of the (+)-M1 metabolites (eg, O-desmethyltramadol) in dogs.[57–60] On the other hand, cats produce O-desmethyltramadol,[61,62] and opioid-induced adverse effects may be observed.

- The formation of the O-desmethyltramadol is produced at much faster rate (3.9-fold) and elimination half-life is longer with higher concentrations of O-desmethyltramadol in cats when compared with dogs.[62,63]

- The half-life of tramadol and the (+)-M1 metabolite is considerably shorter in dogs when compared with humans (2 hours vs 7 hours, respectively). Therefore, intervals of administration would be much shorter in canine individuals than in humans (ie, 4–6 times a day),[64,65] making treatment difficult and limiting clinical use.

---

metabolism and genetic polymorphisms in CYP450 subfamilies. For example, the effects of tramadol can be significantly different depending on the efficiency and amount of a specific CYP450 enzyme among individuals. These differences in CYP450 phenotypes will affect the speed of metabolism and the rate of accumulation or elimination, leading to analgesic failure or effectiveness and the potential for adverse effects. Some human medical centers now use computer clinical decision support with pharmacogenomics tools to guide treatment with tramadol.[66] This is ultimately based on the individual's pharmacogenomics (ie, extensive, intermediate, or poor metabolizers) to predict the safety and efficacy of therapy.

Clinical Use

Tramadol is commonly administered for the treatment of acute and chronic pain. It is often prescribed for long-term postoperative pain. Tramadol is a Schedule IV substance per the Drug Enforcement Agency in the United States because it has potential for abuse. The injectable formulation is used in perioperative pain management in parts of Europe and Latin America, whereas the oral formulation is mostly prescribed in North America, Oceania, and other countries in Europe. Published dosage regimens are variable in dogs and cats. Injectable tramadol (2–4 mg/kg intramuscular) is often used in combination with acepromazine in the premedication of dogs and cats. Doses of 4 to 10 mg/kg orally every 6 hours have been administered in dogs. Doses of 4 mg/kg every 6 hours orally are recommended in cats. Lower doses have been used in the treatment of feline osteoarthritis (2–4 mg/kg orally every 12 hours).[67] The clinical analgesic effects of tramadol have been a subject of substantial controversy in dogs and the causes are described in **Box 8**.

Long-term administration of tramadol produces gastrointestinal adverse effects in some individuals and sedation is commonly observed in cats.[69] Oral formulations are rarely palatable and administration using this route can be an important issue in cats. Cats may salivate profusely after drug administration and therefore treatment compliance is poor. The problem is even more aggravating when dealing with compounded drugs in which quality control and evidence of effects are almost inexistent.

> **Box 8**
> **The controversy involving the analgesic effects of tramadol in dogs**
>
> - Dogs produce much lower concentrations of O-desmethyltramadol than other species. This metabolite is responsible for the opioid analgesic effect after the administration of tramadol.
> - There is usually high individual variability in resulting plasma concentrations of the metabolites of tramadol in dogs and cats.
> - Tramadol has failed to provide analgesia and antinociception in dogs in several studies (see evidence of tramadol in veterinary medicine).
> - Other studies have shown an analgesic effect in the treatment of canine acute pain. However, it must be considered that pain assessment was not always performed by experienced individuals or using validated pain scoring tools, and tramadol was often given in combination with another analgesic drug.
> - Some studies on the use of tramadol in dogs and cats have been criticized because of poor study methodology, inappropriate dosage regimens, lack of control groups and valid models for evaluating clinical pain or antinociception, low sample size, and factors that could have biased the results.
> - Beyond all the controversy, the question remains: does tramadol have a place in canine pain management when administered in combination with NSAIDs or other nonopioid analgesic techniques when compared with these drugs administered alone?[68] The serotoninergic and noradrenergic analgesic effects produced by tramadol might produce some level of clinical analgesia that investigators have not been able to address yet. Until then, the administration of tramadol should be very judicious in dogs, with clear understanding of these limitations, and the drug should never be administered alone for pain management in dogs.

The risk of serotonin toxicity should not be underestimated after the administration of tramadol, especially in combination with other drugs with serotoninergic effects such as other serotonin inhibitors (eg, fluoxetine and trazodone), monoamine oxidase inhibitors (eg, selegiline), and tricyclic antidepressants (eg, amitriptyline and clomipramine). This has been reported in cats and clinical signs include increased neuromuscular activity, tachycardia, fever, tachypnea, and agitation.[70]

Evidence in Humans Related to Pain

Two Cochrane meta-analyses showed that tramadol has good efficacy in the treatment of neuropathic pain and pain-induced osteoarthritis.[71,72] Some evidence also exists for the treatment of low back pain[73]; however, the use of tramadol for the treatment of acute and postoperative pain is not clear.[74] Owing to species differences in drug metabolism (**Box 7**), extrapolation from evidence in humans for veterinary use is not recommended.

Evidence in Veterinary Medicine

Tramadol failed to produce analgesia or antinociception in the canine literature, including in dogs with osteoarthritis.[75] The drug alone did not provide adequate postoperative analgesia in dogs undergoing tibial plateau-leveling osteotomy.[76,77] Nonsteroidal antiinflammatory drugs and pure μ-opioid receptor agonists provided better analgesia than tramadol in dogs undergoing orthopedic and ophthalmic procedures.[78,79] The nonopioid mechanisms of action of tramadol produced limited antinociception in an acute pain model in dogs.[58] Therefore, the overall literature has failed to demonstrate that tramadol should be administered alone for canine acute and chronic pain management. Injectable tramadol has been administered to dogs undergoing soft tissue procedures such as ovariohysterectomy, castration, and unilateral mastectomy.[80–82] Half of dogs undergoing ovariohysterectomy required an intravenous bolus of fentanyl owing to insufficient intraoperative analgesia after tramadol.[80] Tramadol alone did not modulate increases in cerebrocortical activity during castration when compared with morphine.[81]

Tramadol produced some analgesic effects in dogs in a limited number of canine studies.[82] Increases in mechanical nociceptive thresholds were recorded at the 5-hour and 6-hour time points after a single dose of oral tramadol at 9.9 mg/kg in dogs.[59]

Tramadol may be a useful drug for acute and chronic pain in cats. Antinociception and analgesia have been reported after oral and parenteral administration of tramadol in this species.[83–86] Parenteral administration of tramadol provided greater analgesia in cats undergoing ovariohysterectomy when compared with μ-opioid receptor agonist meperidine.[84] However, its oral palatability and dosing intervals often preclude its oral administration in feline practice. Analgesic failure has been reported after the administration of tramadol in cats, and signs of pain should be monitored.[83]

REFERENCES

1. Cheng J-K, Chiou L-C. Mechanisms of the antinociceptive action of gabapentin. J Pharmacol Sci 2006;100(5):471–86.

2. Hayashida K-I, Eisenach JC. Descending noradrenergic inhibition: an important mechanism of gabapentin analgesia in neuropathic pain. Adv Exp Med Biol 2018;1099:93–100.

3. Hayashida K-I, Obata H. Strategies to treat chronic pain and strengthen impaired descending noradrenergic inhibitory system. Int J Mol Sci 2019;20(4) [pii:E822].

4. Radulovic L, Türck D, Von Hodenberg A, et al. Disposition of gabapentin (Neurotin) in mice, rats, dogs and monkeys. Drug Metab Dispos 1995;23(4):441–8.

5. Adrian D, Papich M, Baynes R, et al. Pharmacokinetics of gabapentin in cats. J Vet Intern Med 2018;32:1996–2002.

6. Siao KT, Pypendop BH, Ilkiw JE. Pharmacokinetics of gabapentin in cats. Am J Vet Res 2010;71(7):817–21.

7. Kukanich B, Cohen R. Pharmacokinetics of oral gabapentin in greyhound dogs. J Vet Pharmacol Ther 2011;187(1):133–5.

8. Vollmer KO, von Hodenberg A, Kolle EU. Pharmacokinetics and metabolism of gabapentin in rat, dog and man. Arzneimittelforschung 1986;36(5):830–9.

9. Aghighi SA, Tipold A, Piechotta M, et al. Assessment of the effects of adjunctive gabapentin on postoperative pain after intervertebral disc surgery in dogs. Vet Anaesth Analg 2012;39(6):636–46.

10. Crociolli GC, Cassu RN, Barbero RC, et al. Gabapentin as an adjuvant for postoperative pain management in dogs undergoing mastectomy. J Vet Med Sci 2015;77(8):1011–5.

11. Steagall PV, Benito J, Monteiro BP, et al. Analgesic effects of gabapentin and buprenorphine in cats undergoing ovariohysterectomy using two pain-scoring systems: a randomized clinical trial. J Feline Med Surg 2018;20(8):741–8.

12. Wagner AE, Mich PM, Uhrig SR, et al. Clinical evaluation of perioperative administration of gabapentin as an adjunct for postoperative analgesia in dogs undergoing amputation of a forelimb. J Am Vet Med Assoc 2010;236(7):751–6.

13. Pankratz KE, Ferris KK, Griffith EH, et al. Use of single-dose oral gabapentin to attenuate fear responses in cage-trap confined community cats: a double-blind, placebo-controlled field trial. J Feline Med Surg 2018;20(6):535–43.

14. van Haaften K, Eichstadt Forsythe L, Stelow E, et al. Effects of a single preappointment dose of gabapentin on signs of stress in cats during transportation and veterinary examination. J Am Vet Med Assoc 2017;251(10):1175–81.
15. Hu J, Huang D, Li M, et al. Effects of a single dose of preoperative pregabalin and gabapentin for acute postoperative pain: a network meta-analysis of randomized controlled trials. J Pain Res 2018;11:2633–43.
16. Felder L, Saccone G, Scuotto S, et al. Perioperative gabapentin and post cesarean pain control: a systematic review and meta-analysis of randomized controlled trials. Eur J Obstet Gynecol Reprod Biol 2019;233:98–106.
17. Zeng M, Dong J, Lin N, et al. Preoperative gabapentin administration improves acute postoperative analgesia in patients undergoing craniotomy: a randomized controlled trial. J Neurosurg Anesthesiol 2018. [Epub ahead of print].
18. Li X-D, Han C, Yu W-L. Is gabapentin effective and safe in open hysterectomy? A PRISMA compliant meta-analysis of randomized controlled trials. J Clin Anesth 2017;41:76–83.
19. Moskowitz EE, Garabedian L, Harden K, et al. A double-blind, randomized controlled trial of gabapentin vs. placebo for acute pain management in critically ill patients with rib fractures. Injury 2018;49(9):1693–8.
20. Tulandi T, Krishnamurthy S, Mansour F, et al. A triple-blind randomized trial of preemptive use of gabapentin before laparoscopic hysterectomy for benign gynaecologic conditions. J Obstet Gynaecol Can 2019 [pii:S1701-2163(18)30930-30937].
21. Verret M, Lauzier F, Zarychanski R, et al. Perioperative use of gabapentinoids for the management of postoperative acute pain: protocol of a systematic review and meta- analysis. Syst Rev 2019;8:24.
22. Chou R, Gordon DB, de Leon-casasola OA, et al. Management of postoperative pain: a clinical practice guideline from the American Pain Society, the American Society of Regional Anesthesia and Pain Medicine, and the American Society of Anesthesiologists' Committee on Regional Anesthesia, Executive Committee, and Administrative Council. J Pain 2016;17(2):131–57.
23. Mathews K, Kronen PW, Lascelles D, et al. Guidelines for recognition, assessment and treatment of pain: WSAVA Global Pain Council members and co-authors of this document. J Small Anim Pract 2014;55:E10–68.
24. Cashmore R, Harcourt-Brown T, Freeman P, et al. Clinical diagnosis and treatment of suspected neuropathic pain in three dogs. Aust Vet J 2009; 87(February):45–50.
25. KuKanich B. Outpatient oral analgesics in dogs and cats beyond nonsteroidal antiinflammatory drugs. An evidence-based approach. Vet Clin North Am Small Anim Pract 2013;43(5):1109–25.
26. Steagall PVM, Monteiro-steagall BP. Multimodal analgesia for perioperative pain in three cats. J Feline Med Surg 2013;15(8):737–43.
27. Vettorato E, Corletto F. Gabapentin as part of multi-modal analgesia in two cats suffering multiple injuries. Vet Anaesth Analg 2011;38(5):518–20.
28. Lorenz ND, Comerford EJ, Iff I. Long-term use of gabapentin for musculoskeletal disease and trauma in three cats. J Feline Med Surg 2012;15(6):507–12.
29. Reid P, Pypendop BH, Ilkiw JE. The effects of intravenous gabapentin administration on the minimum alveolar concentration of isoflurane in cats. J Anesth Analg 2010;111(3):633–7.
30. Pypendop BH, Siao KT, Ilkiw JE. Thermal antinociceptive effect of orally administered gabapentin in healthy cats. Am J Vet Res 2010;71(9):8–13.

31. Ebert B, Mikkelsen S, Thorkildsen C, et al. Norketamine, the main metabolite of ketamine, is a non-competitive NMDA receptor antagonist in the rat cortex and spinal cord. Eur J Pharmacol 1997;333(1):99–104.

32. Pozzi A, Muir WW, Traverso F. Prevention of central sensitization and pain by N-methyl-D-aspartate receptor antagonists. J Am Vet Med Assoc 2006;228(1): 53–60.

33. McNicol ED, Schumann R, Haroutounian S. A systematic review and meta-analysis of ketamine for the prevention of persistent post-surgical pain. Acta Anaesthesiol Scand 2014;58(10):1199–213.

34. Bell RF, Dahl JB, Moore RA, et al. Peri-operative ketamine for acute post-operative pain: a quantitative and qualitative systematic review (Cochrane review). Acta Anaesthesiol Scand 2005;49(10):1405–28.

35. Shapiro J, Jersky J, Katzav S, et al. Anesthetic drugs accelerate the progression of postoperative metastases of mouse tumors. J Clin Invest 1981;68(3):678–85.

36. Kim R. Effects of surgery and anesthetic choice on immunosuppression and cancer recurrence. J Transl Med 2018;16(1):8.

37. Melamed R, Bar-Yosef S, Shakhar G, et al. Suppression of natural killer cell activity and promotion of tumor metastasis by ketamine, thiopental, and halothane, but not by propofol: mediating mechanisms and prophylactic measures. Anesth Analg 2003;97(5):1331–9.

38. Beilin B, Bessler H, Mayburd E, et al. Effects of preemptive analgesia on pain and cytokine production in the postoperative period. Anesthesiology 2003;98(1): 151–5.

39. Zhou N, Fu Z, Li H, et al. Ketamine, as adjuvant analgesics for patients with refractory cancer pain, does affect IL-2/IFN-gamma expression of T cells in vitro?: a prospective, randomized, double-blind study. Medicine (Baltimore) 2017;96(16):e6639.

40. Kawasaki C, Kawasaki T, Ogata M, et al. Ketamine isomers suppress superantigen-induced proinflammatory cytokine production in human whole blood. Can J Anaesth 2001;48(8):819–23.

41. Kehlet H, Dahl JB. The value of "multimodal" or "balanced analgesia" in postoperative pain treatment. Anesth Analg 1993;77(5):1048–56.

42. Sarrau S, Jourdan J, Dupuis-Soyris F, et al. Effects of postoperative ketamine infusion on pain control and feeding behaviour in bitches undergoing mastectomy. J Small Anim Pract 2007;48(12):670–6.

43. Wagner AE, Walton JA, Hellyer PW, et al. Use of low doses of ketamine administered by constant rate infusion as an adjunct for postoperative analgesia in dogs. J Am Vet Med Assoc 2002;221(1):72–5.

44. Gutierrez-Blanco E, Victoria-Mora JM, Ibancovichi-Camarillo JA, et al. Postoperative analgesic effects of either a constant rate infusion of fentanyl, lidocaine, ketamine, dexmedetomidine, or the combination lidocaine-ketamine-dexmedetomidine after ovariohysterectomy in dogs. Vet Anaesth Analg 2015; 42(3):309–18.

45. Boscan P, Pypendop BH, Solano AM, et al. Cardiovascular and respiratory effects of ketamine infusions in isoflurane-anesthetized dogs before and during noxious stimulation. Am J Vet Res 2005;66(12):2122–9.

46. Gutierrez-Blanco E, Victoria-Mora JM, Ibancovichi-Camarillo JA, et al. Evaluation of the isoflurane-sparing effects of fentanyl, lidocaine, ketamine, dexmedetomidine, or the combination lidocaine-ketamine-dexmedetomidine during ovariohysterectomy in dogs. Vet Anaesth Analg 2013;40(6):599–609.

47. Pypendop BH, Solano A, Boscan P, et al. Characteristics of the relationship between plasma ketamine concentration and its effect on the minimum alveolar concentration of isoflurane in dogs. Vet Anaesth Analg 2007;34(3):209–12.
48. Cohen SP, Bhatia A, Buvanendran A, et al. Consensus guidelines on the use of intravenous ketamine infusions for chronic pain from the American Society of Regional Anesthesia and Pain Medicine, the American Academy of Pain Medicine, and the American Society of Anesthesiologists. Reg Anesth Pain Med 2018;43(5):521–46.
49. Slingsby LS, Waterman-Pearson AE. The post-operative analgesic effects of ketamine after canine ovariohysterectomy–a comparison between pre- or post-operative administration. Res Vet Sci 2000;69(2):147–52.
50. Love L, Egger C, Rohrbach B, et al. The effect of ketamine on the MACBAR of sevoflurane in dogs. Vet Anaesth Analg 2011;38(4):292–300.
51. Muir WW 3rd, Wiese AJ, March PA. Effects of morphine, lidocaine, ketamine, and morphine-lidocaine-ketamine drug combination on minimum alveolar concentration in dogs anesthetized with isoflurane. Am J Vet Res 2003;64(9):1155–60.
52. Pascoe PJ, Ilkiw JE, Craig C, et al. The effects of ketamine on the minimum alveolar concentration of isoflurane in cats. Vet Anaesth Analg 2007;34(1):31–9.
53. Solano AM, Pypendop BH, Boscan PL, et al. Effect of intravenous administration of ketamine on the minimum alveolar concentration of isoflurane in anesthetized dogs. Am J Vet Res 2006;67(1):21–5.
54. Steagall PVM, Aucoin M, Monteiro BP, et al. Clinical effects of a constant rate infusion of remifentanil, alone or in combination with ketamine, in cats anesthetized with isoflurane. J Am Vet Med Assoc 2015;246(9):976–81.
55. Grond S, Sablotzki A. Clinical pharmacology of tramadol. Clin Pharmacokinet 2004;43(13):879–923.
56. Perez Jimenez TE, Mealey KL, Schnider D, et al. Identification of canine cytochrome P-450s (CYPs) metabolizing the tramadol (+)-M1 and (+)-M2 metabolites to the tramadol (+)-M5 metabolite in dog liver microsomes. J Vet Pharmacol Ther 2018;41(6):815–24.
57. Benitez ME, Roush JK, KuKanich B, et al. Pharmacokinetics of hydrocodone and tramadol administered for control of postoperative pain in dogs following tibial plateau leveling osteotomy. Am J Vet Res 2015;76(9):763–70.
58. Kogel B, Terlinden R, Schneider J. Characterisation of tramadol, morphine and tapentadol in an acute pain model in Beagle dogs. Vet Anaesth Analg 2014; 41(3):297–304.
59. Kukanich B, Papich MG. Pharmacokinetics and antinociceptive effects of oral tramadol hydrochloride administration in Greyhounds. Am J Vet Res 2011;72(2): 256–62.
60. Vettorato E, Zonca A, Isola M, et al. Pharmacokinetics and efficacy of intravenous and extradural tramadol in dogs. Vet J 2010;183(3):310–5.
61. Cagnardi P, Villa R, Zonca A, et al. Pharmacokinetics, intraoperative effect and postoperative analgesia of tramadol in cats. Res Vet Sci 2011;90(3):503–9.
62. Pypendop BH, Ilkiw JE. Pharmacokinetics of tramadol, and its metabolite O-desmethyl-tramadol, in cats. J Vet Pharmacol Ther 2008;31(1):52–9.
63. Perez Jimenez T, Mealey K, Grubb T, et al. Tramadol metabolism to O-desmethyl tramadol (M1) and N-desmethyl tramadol (M2) by dog liver microsomes: Species comparison and identification of responsible canine cytochrome P-450s (CYPs). Drug Metab Dispos 2016;44(12):1963–72.
64. KuKanich B, Papich MG. Pharmacokinetics of tramadol and the metabolite O-desmethyltramadol in dogs. J Vet Pharmacol Ther 2004;27(4):239–46.

65. Wu WN, McKown LA, Gauthier AD, et al. Metabolism of the analgesic drug, tramadol hydrochloride, in rat and dog. Xenobiotica 2001;31(7):423–41.
66. Miotto K, Cho AK, Khalil MA, et al. Trends in tramadol: pharmacology, metabolism, and misuse. Anesth Analg 2017;124(1):44–51.
67. Monteiro BP, Klinck MP, Moreau M, et al. Analgesic efficacy of tramadol in cats with naturally occurring osteoarthritis. PLoS One 2017;12(4):e0175565.
68. Flor PB, Yazbek KVB, Ida KK, et al. Tramadol plus metamizole combined or not with anti-inflammatory drugs is clinically effective for moderate to severe chronic pain treatment in cancer patients. Vet Anaesth Analg 2013;40(3):316–27.
69. Guedes AGP, Meadows JM, Pypendop BH, et al. Evaluation of tramadol for treatment of osteoarthritis in geriatric cats. J Am Vet Med Assoc 2018;252(5):565–71.
70. Indrawirawan Y, McAlees T. Tramadol toxicity in a cat: case report and literature review of serotonin syndrome. J Feline Med Surg 2014;16(7):572–8.
71. Cepeda MS, Camargo F, Zea C, et al. Tramadol for osteoarthritis. Cochrane Database Syst Rev 2006;(3):CD005522.
72. Duehmke RM, Derry S, Wiffen PJ, et al. Tramadol for neuropathic pain in adults. Cochrane Database Syst Rev 2017;(6):CD003726.
73. Chaparro LE, Furlan AD, Deshpande A, et al. Opioids compared to placebo or other treatments for chronic low-back pain. Cochrane Database Syst Rev 2013;(8):CD004959.
74. Sonis J. Tramadol for acute pain: a review of the evidence. Am Fam Physician 2005;72(10):1964 [author reply: 1964, 1966].
75. Budsberg SC, Torres BT, Kleine SA, et al. Lack of effectiveness of tramadol hydrochloride for the treatment of pain and joint dysfunction in dogs with chronic osteoarthritis. J Am Vet Med Assoc 2018;252(4):427–32.
76. Davila D, Keeshen TP, Evans RB, et al. Comparison of the analgesic efficacy of perioperative firocoxib and tramadol administration in dogs undergoing tibial plateau leveling osteotomy. J Am Vet Med Assoc 2013;243(2):225–31.
77. Benitez ME, Roush JK, McMurphy R, et al. Clinical efficacy of hydrocodone-acetaminophen and tramadol for control of postoperative pain in dogs following tibial plateau leveling osteotomy. Am J Vet Res 2015;76(9):755–62.
78. Cardozo LB, Cotes LC, Kahvegian MAP, et al. Evaluation of the effects of methadone and tramadol on postoperative analgesia and serum interleukin-6 in dogs undergoing orthopaedic surgery. BMC Vet Res 2014;10:194.
79. Delgado C, Bentley E, Hetzel S, et al. Comparison of carprofen and tramadol for postoperative analgesia in dogs undergoing enucleation. J Am Vet Med Assoc 2014;245(12):1375–81.
80. Kongara K, Chambers JP, Johnson CB. Effects of tramadol, morphine or their combination in dogs undergoing ovariohysterectomy on peri-operative electroencephalographic responses and post-operative pain. N Z Vet J 2012;60(2):129–35.
81. Kongara K, Chambers JP, Johnson CB, et al. Effects of tramadol or morphine in dogs undergoing castration on intra-operative electroencephalogram responses and post-operative pain. N Z Vet J 2013;61(6):349–53.
82. Teixeira RC, Monteiro ER, Campagnol D, et al. Effects of tramadol alone, in combination with meloxicam or dipyrone, on postoperative pain and the analgesic requirement in dogs undergoing unilateral mastectomy with or without ovariohysterectomy. Vet Anaesth Analg 2013;40(6):641–9.
83. Brondani JT, Loureiro Luna SP, Beier SL, et al. Analgesic efficacy of perioperative use of vedaprofen, tramadol or their combination in cats undergoing ovariohysterectomy. J Feline Med Surg 2009;11(6):420–9.

84. Evangelista MC, Silva RA, Cardozo LB, et al. Comparison of preoperative trama-dol and pethidine on postoperative pain in cats undergoing ovariohysterectomy. BMC Vet Res 2014;10:252.
85. Pypendop BH, Siao KT, Ilkiw JE. Effects of tramadol hydrochloride on the thermal threshold in cats. Am J Vet Res 2009;70(12):1465–70.
86. Steagall PVM, Taylor PM, Brondani JT, et al. Antinociceptive effects of tramadol and acepromazine in cats. J Feline Med Surg 2008;10(1):24–31.

Rehabilitation Therapy in Perioperative Pain Management

Molly J. Flaherty, DVM, CCRP

KEYWORDS

- Veterinary rehabilitation • Cryotherapy • Electrical stimulation
- Pulsed electromagnetic therapy • Laser therapy • Pain management • Analgesia
- Opioids

KEY POINTS

- Research indicates that a variety of modalities used in veterinary rehabilitation provide effective analgesia and can reduce the use of opioids in postoperative recovery.
- Cryotherapy, pulsed electromagnetic field therapy (PEMF), transcutaneous electrical nerve stimulation, and laser therapy used in veterinary rehabilitation can have benefits to perioperative pain management.
- These modalities can safely be incorporated into the clinic surgical pain management protocol, and pet owners can continue cryotherapy and PEMF in home.
- Additional clinical studies in veterinary medicine are needed to evaluate the effectiveness of these modalities in reducing the need for opioids in veterinary patients.

INTRODUCTION

Rehabilitation therapy incorporates many physical modalities that can be used to reduce postsurgical pain. There is ample evidence showing cryotherapy, pulsed electromagnetic field therapy (PEMF), transcutaneous electrical nerve stimulation (TENS), and laser therapy can be used to reduce pain and inflammation. In accordance, a growing number of studies show that the use of these as adjunctive treatments to pharmacotherapy can optimize pain control and reduce the need for pain medications, including opioids.

Veterinarians are continually seeking means of analgesia that may help reduce the need of pharmaceuticals, including opioids. Noninvasive nonpharmacologic methods of pain control contribute to reducing side effects and provide opioid-sparing options.

Disclosures: None declared.
Department of Clinical Science, Ryan Veterinary Hospital of the University of Pennsylvania, 3900 Delancey Street, Philadelphia, PA 19104, USA
E-mail address: MollyFL@UPenn.edu

An understanding of the evidence, effects, applications, and contraindications will guide practitioners on the modalities they may want to incorporate into their surgical pain management protocols.

CRYOTHERAPY

Application of cold therapy is known to produce vasoconstriction, which decreases local blood flow, inflammatory response, and edema, thereby reducing pain. Skin and underlying tissue temperatures can be decreased to a depth of 2 to 4 cm.[1,2] Anesthetic effects can be achieved through slowing of nerve conduction velocity and increasing pain thresholds.[3] Cooling of muscle tissue also decreases muscle spasms, possibly because of a cooling effect on decreasing muscle spindle activity.[4]

Cold therapy has widely been used for both acute and chronic musculoskeletal and postsurgical pain. Controlled studies have found reduced levels of pain in human patients receiving cryotherapy for postoperative joint[5,6] and spine surgery[7] and dentistry root canal treatment.[8] A decrease in human patient opioid use with cryotherapy treatment during the postoperative period has been shown in randomized controlled studies.[7,9] It is plausible that the same would be true for animal patients, although other effective methods of measuring opioid need would have to be considered.

Recommendations are to apply cryotherapy 2 to 4 times daily for 20 minutes for the first 3 to 4 days after surgery.[10] Methods of application most commonly used in veterinary patients include cool packs, ice massage, and cold compression therapy.

Ice Packs

Ice pack are the most frequently used method, involving a freezer bag of crushed ice or a gel pack that has been cooled in a freezer. A towel or cloth should be placed between the patient and the ice pack to prevent skin damage. Application is typically 15 to 20 minutes 3 to 6 times per day.

Ice Massage

Paper cups may be filled with water and frozen. The ice can be directly applied to skin surface in a continuous circular method for 5 to 10 minutes (**Fig. 1**). Ice massage was found to reach lower muscle tissue temperature more quickly than with ice bag application, although both were effective in decreasing intramuscular temperature.[11]

Cold Compression Therapy

This method allows cold therapy to be combined with compression. Several commercial units for veterinary use are available. Wraps are applied over the affected limb or joint that have been designed to fit small animals (**Fig. 2**). This technique is particularly effective following orthopedic surgery. Following knee surgery in human patients, cold compress therapy was found to have improved results compared with cryotherapy alone in pain scores in the first 24 hours and in decrease in swelling in the first 48 hours.[12] In canine patients, following extracapsular repair of cranial cruciate ligament rupture, cold compression decreased soft tissue swelling in the first 72 hours with or without bandaging compared with bandaging alone.[13] Another canine study found decreased signs of pain, swelling, and lameness and increased range of motion with cryotherapy compared with no cryotherapy treatment in the first 24 hours after tibial plateau–leveling osteotomy surgery.[14]

Cryotherapy is a safe and low-cost method of pain relief that can easily be incorporated in postoperative pain management and potentially reduces the need for pharmaceuticals, including narcotics. It is generally well tolerated by animal patients. Various

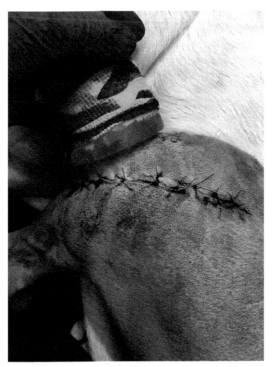

Fig. 1. Ice massage to relieve postoperative inflammation and edema.

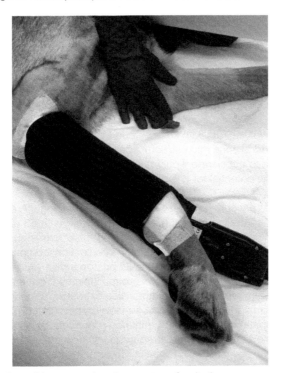

Fig. 2. Postoperative cold compression therapy to a forelimb.

studies in humans have shown that there is effective decrease of skin temperature when cryotherapy is applied over plaster and synthetic casts[15,16] and light bandages.[17] However, cold therapy over Robert Jones bandages (RJBs) was less effective.[16] Thus patients in which an RJB is applied should receive cryotherapy before application of the bandage. Side effects and contraindications are minimal. Use should be avoided over areas of ischemia and open wounds, and skin should be checked every 5 minutes for tissue damage.

PULSED ELECTROMAGNETIC FIELD THERAPY

PEMF uses a device that transmits a nonthermal electromagnetic field that is applied over areas of pain to decrease inflammation. The commercially available units have variable specifications for the intended mechanism of action or treatment target. The targeted PEMF (tPEMF) devices for pain relief are configured to increase intracellular Ca^{2+}, which leads to increased calcium binding to calmodulin. This process leads to a variety of downstream pathways, including the production of nitric oxide.[18,19] Evidence supports that tPEMF effects depend on nitric oxide cascades. Nitric oxide can reduce inflammation through increase in blood and lymph flow reducing pain and edema.[20]

PEMF treatment has been used since the 1970s for treatment of nonhealing bone fractures in humans.[21] The US Food and Drug Administration (FDA) cleared targeted PEMF devices for treatment of postoperative pain and edema. There is a growing amount of research evidence that PEMF is a safe, noninvasive, and effective modality for postoperative pain control, inflammation reduction, and tissue healing.

Studies have shown that postoperative use of PEMF for pain relief in human patients reduced the amount of pain medication used.[19,20,22–24] Of these studies, 2 were double-blinded, placebo-controlled studies with human breast reconstruction patients, which found significant reductions in postoperative pain scores of 2.0-fold[23] and 2.2-fold[19] as well as reduction of narcotic use by patients for pain management. It can be theorized that the use of PEMF in the perioperative period in animal patients could also reduce the need for analgesics, including opioids.

Studies using PEMF for pain in human patients have also found it safe and effective for low back pain,[25,26] dental pain,[27] and for pain management of knee osteoarthritis.[28] A study involving rats with knee osteoarthritis suggests that PEMF treatment preserved subchondral bone microstructure compared with control.[29] PEMF has also been shown in rats to accelerate would healing by increasing tensile strength.[30] This finding indicates the potential for a wide range of PEMF use in pain management and healing.

Studies in animal patients have also had supportive findings. A double-blind, randomized, placebo-controlled clinical trial was performed with 53 client-owned dogs following hemilaminectomy for natural occurring disk extrusion. Dogs receiving PEMF had reduced owner-administered pain medication compared with a sham group and improved wound scores at 6 weeks postoperative. Codeine was administered 1.8 times more frequently in the sham group.[31] In canine patients with paraplegia and loss of nociception from thoracolumbar disc extrusion, a randomized, placebo-controlled, clinical trial found PEMF reduced incision-associated pain after recovery and may reduce spinal cord injury and enhance proprioceptive placing. Treatments were started at the time of surgical preparation and continued every 2 hours for 2 weeks and then twice daily for 4 weeks. Treatment group identity was masked from clinicians, technicians, and pet owners. Over a 6-week period, higher pain thresholds were found in PEMF-treated dogs compared with placebo. This study showed a significant effect on postoperative pain management.[32] A randomized controlled clinical trial evaluating postoperative pain management with PEMF following ovariohysterectomy in dogs concluded that, although there was no clear benefit, it may reduce postsurgical pain and augment morphine analgesia in canine patients.[33] In dogs with osteoarthritis, a controlled study found dogs receiving PEMF performed better in gait analysis and owner assessment compared with the control group.[34]

Devices commonly used in veterinary medicine are small portable loops that emit the PEMF in an elliptical range around the loop. For treatment they are placed over or around the area of pain, such as over the spine (**Fig. 3**). Some companies offer accessories to hold the device over the desired area. Treatments are generally 15 minutes, starting 3 to 4 times per day. Targeted PEMF treatments are athermal, do not produce sensation, and are well tolerated by animal patients.

PEMF is a painless and convenient way to augment postoperative pain in hospital and continued pain management after discharge in animal patients. No adverse effects were noted in studies.[18,19,22,23,28,30] During one study a canine patient ingested the device, and it is advisable to only be used with direct supervision.[32] One portable PEMF device manufacturer cautions use over tumor site of hemangiosarcoma, because of potential increase in blood flow, and on animals with a pacemaker, because of potential interference.[35]

TRANSCUTANEOUS ELECTRICAL NERVE STIMULATION

TENS is the application of low-voltage electrical impulses through electrodes on the skin using various waveforms, frequencies, and amplitudes. TENS has been used for treatment of painful acute and chronic conditions since the 1970s.[36] Conventional TENS (50 Hz or greater) stimulates large cutaneous Aβ fibers that stimulate inhibitory neurons in the spinal cord dorsal horn, blocking transmission of pain impulses to the brain. This basis of pain control is elucidated by the gate-control theory described by Melzac and Wall.[37]

Several studies indicate the release of endogenous opioids with TENS treatment, particularly at the low frequency settings (10 Hz). Use of local naltrexone in rats blocked the effects of low-frequency and not high-frequency TENS, indicating low-frequency TENS involves the release of endogenous opioids and high-frequency TENS involves a non–opioid-medicated mechanism.[38] Naloxone administration in

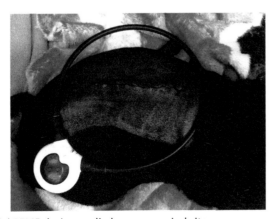

Fig. 3. Commercial PEMF device applied over a surgical site.

the rostral ventral medulla was found to block the antihyperalgesic effects of low-frequency TENS in rats.[39] Antihyperalgesia produced by TENS in arthritic rats was blocked by low doses of naloxone in the spinal cord for low-frequency TENS, whereas high doses of naloxone were needed to produce the same results in high-frequency TENS.[40] These studies suggest that incorporating TENS could decrease the need for opioids in pain management by activating the endogenous opioid system.

Multiple studies in human patients show TENS therapy to be beneficial in pain reduction following surgical procedures.[41–44] These findings are useful in consideration of animal patients. One meta-analysis of randomized placebo-controlled studies on humans from 1966 to 2001 concluded that TENS reduced postoperative pain and analgesic need during the first 3 days after surgery. Optimal dose was found to be 85 Hz for conventional TENS.[45]

When focused on narcotic pain medications, studies have determined a reduced need for opioids when TENS is used postoperatively. Another meta-analysis of randomized controlled studies concluded that TENS treatments (80–150 Hz) could significantly reduce pain and opioid consumption in the first 48 hours after total knee arthroplasty as well as reduce adverse opioid effects in human patients compared with control groups.[46] A double-blind, randomized trial found TENS (150 Hz) decreased pain and opioid use in the immediate postoperative period following arthroscopic rotator cuff repair in human patients. TENS significantly reduced opioid use by more than 25% at 48 hours and 1 week after surgery as well as producing statistically significant reductions in pain scores.[47] Sham controlled studies involving the use of TENS over acupoints in human patients found reduced patient use of postoperative fentanyl following total hip arthoplasty[44] and reduced need of hydromorphone following abdominal surgery.[48] It is plausible to assume the same results could be found in animal patients, resulting in reduced opioid use and reduced side effects of medications.

Application postoperatively involves placement of electrodes parallel to the incision (**Fig. 4**) or on 2 sides of the surgical joint. Electrodes should be at least 2.5 cm (1 inch) apart but not far apart and surrounding the area of pain to allow the electrical current to pass through the painful region.[49] Segmental placement may also be done where electrodes are placed over the nerve root of the spinal segment corresponding with the regional area of pain.

TENS was found to have antihyperalgesia effects when electrodes were placed on the limb contralateral to the injury.[38] This finding suggests that, if a patient is hypersensitive to treatment on the surgical or injured limb, treating the contralateral limb may have the same analgesic effects. High-intensity stimulation, high-frequency TENS is more likely effective for short-term use and should be considered postoperatively, with alternating low and high frequency for chronic use to prevent tolerance.[50] Parameters most frequently used for conventional TENS are high frequency (50–150 Hz) short pulse duration (2–50 μs) and low intensity.[51] These settings are generally more comfortable than low-frequency TENS (1–10 Hz). High-frequency, short pulse duration, conventional TENS settings are appropriate for acute postoperative pain treatment by activation of the gate mechanism for pain control and can easily be incorporated in the postoperative period as an adjunct to pain management protocols. Electrodes are placed over skin where fur has been clipped using contact gel such as ultrasonography gel or, if short fur is present, using enough gel to allow good contact.[52] Intensity should be set at a comfortable sensory level, below the level at which a visible reaction is stimulated, and treatment should last for 10 to 15 minutes and can be repeated as needed 1 to 2 times daily.

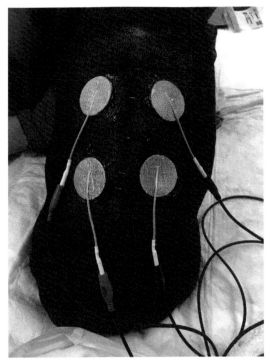

Fig. 4. TENS electrode placement along a surgical incision.

Although there are few side effects known, precautions include areas of impaired sensation or skin damage. Contraindications include directly over the heart, carotid sinus, or over the trunk during pregnancy; in animals with pacemakers or seizure disorders; and over infection, neoplasms, thrombosis, or thrombophlebitis.[51]

LASER THERAPY

Laser is an acronym for light amplification by stimulated emission of radiation. Commonly referred to as photobiomodulation, photons from lasers are absorbed through cytochromes in mitochondria of target cells. This treatment results in increased biological responses, including accelerated ATP production. ATP is necessary for cellular energy production and leads to biological responses that enhance tissue repair and decrease pain and inflammation.[53] Class 3b and class 4 lasers offer the same effects, with class 4 having the ability to deliver more energy per time through higher operational wattage. Both of these are commonly used in veterinary practices for pain management and healing and are well tolerated by animal patients (**Fig. 5**).

Variable wavelengths are used in therapy lasers. Wavelengths between 800 and 1100 nm are able to penetrate deep tissue and stimulate photobiomodulation.[54] More commonly, wavelengths of 810 nm to 980 nm are used for pain management. Dose of laser applied to treatment area is measured in energy density (J/cm^2). Dosages used can vary greatly depending on the specific unit, condition, and species being treated. An author in 1 veterinary publication has found it beneficial to start therapeutic laser treatment during surgery intraoperatively at 3 to 4 J/cm^2 at no more than 4 W power following aseptic technique.[55] Postoperative treatment

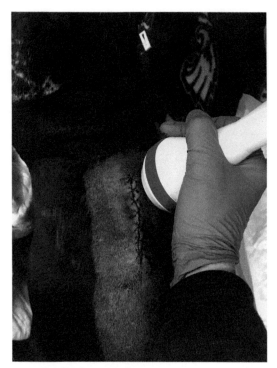

Fig. 5. Laser therapy application in surgical recovery.

recommendations typically are from 1 to 4 J/cm^2 for acute postsurgical pain and inflammation.

Laser has many therapeutic applications in veterinary medicine, including resolution of edema, wound and incision healing, muscle strain, ligament and tendon injury, minimizing inflammation, reduction of inflammation, nerve regrowth, and acute or chronic pain management. These applications can benefit patients in healing and pain reduction in the perioperative period. It has been postulated that photomedicine can reduce the need of opioids and potential drug abuse.[56]

There is compiling research evidence supporting laser use for decreasing pain and inflammation[57–63]; in wound healing[64–67] through increased granulation tissue,[68] collagen fibers,[69] and fibroblasts[70]; and in strength of repairing ligaments.[71] Laser treatment has been found to inhibit prostaglandin E_2[59,61] production and promote analgesic effects through endogenous opioid mechanisms. Several studies in rats have shown that analgesia produced by laser treatment was partially or transiently reversed by naloxone administration.[62,64,72] A study in mice found laser treatment reduced naloxone-induced morphine withdrawal symptoms.[73] These findings indicate that laser has effects through the endogenous opioid mechanism.

A retrospective literature review found evidence supporting the use of laser for pain, postulating that this could be a more safe and cost-effective alternative to opioids in human patients.[60] A randomized clinical trial with 54 human patients following tibial fracture surgery found reduced pain and significantly less opioid use in the laser-treated patients in the first 24 hours following surgery. Patients were treated with laser once postoperatively at 9 J/cm^2 around the joint, and muscle trigger points were treated with 4 J/cm^2.[74]

In canine patients, laser treatment over the hemilaminectomy site daily for 5 days, dosed at 2 to 8 J/cm^2, was found to decrease the time to ambulation following acute T3-L3 intervertebral disc rupture compared with a control group.[75] Pain control effects of laser were not evaluated in this study and the reasons for improved time to ambulation could be postulated to be from decrease in pain and increase in nerve regeneration. A randomized, blind, placebo-controlled trial involving 20 dogs with elbow osteoarthritis found more than 50% reduction in nonsteroidal antiinflammatory drug dose required to control pain in laser-treated dogs compared with 0% reduction in the sham group dogs. Laser was dosed at 10 to 20 J/cm^2 twice weekly for 2 weeks.[76] In 20 feline patients, a randomized controlled study, using laser at 3 J/cm^2 over acupuncture points before ovariohysterectomy, found reduced postoperative analgesic need in the patients receiving laser acupuncture compared with control patients.[77] Laser being applied to acupuncture points may recruit other means of pain relief than direct inflammation reduction. Another study involved 12 canine patients randomly assigned to laser treatment or control following tibial plateau–leveling osteotomy. This study found no beneficial effects of laser in function or reducing pain. Laser treatment was dosed at 1.5 to 2.25 J/cm^2 and administered postoperatively and through 8 weeks of recovery.[78] The investigators postulate the lack of established protocols for veterinary patients as a limitation to guidance for protocol.

The variable specification in units used and dosages administered makes comparison of studies difficult. Solidification of guidelines and standardization of protocols are still lacking. More research and consensus are needed in the optimal dosages for specific uses in each species. Lower dosages may not be effective and higher dosages may inhibit recovery or damage tissues. Multiple dosages at higher doses could be inhibitory[70] because of potential cellular damage, which could prolong recovery time and impede pain management following surgery. Recommended treatment settings for animals set by the manufacturer for each unit should generally be used.

Laser treatment is effective, noninvasive, and easily tolerated by animal patients. Biostimulation lasers are cleared by the FDA for use in pain relief. As an adjunct analgesic method for patients in the perioperative period, laser should be considered a viable option to control pain, reduce the need for opioids, and consequently reduce side effects. Laser providers should be well trained in safe laser administration and familiar with the appropriate application of the specific unit they are using. Precautions include wearing protective eyewear to prevent retinal damage and prevention of overheating tissues. Contraindicated areas of treatment to be aware of are over neoplasia, pregnant uterus, gonads, cornea, active bleeding, endocrine glands, and active epiphyses.

SUMMARY

Physical modalities can be effective in perioperative analgesia for reducing pain and inflammation in veterinary patients. Use of these therapies can contribute to reduction of pharmaceutical medication use, including opioids, and decrease potential side effects. Use of these modalities synergistically with traditional pharmacotherapy can maximize pain management in recovery. Knowledge of the effects, methods of application, precautions, and adverse effects is important for proper use and maximal benefits.

REFERENCES

1. Millis DL. Physical therapy and rehabilitation. In: Gaynor JS, Muir WW, editors. Veterinary pain management. 3rd edition. St Louis (MO): Elsevier; 2015. p. 383–421.

2. Niebaum K, McCauley L, Medina C. Rehabilitation physical modalities. In: Zink C, Van Dyke JB, editors. Canine sports medicine and rehabilitation. 2nd edition. Hoboken (NJ): Wiley Blackwell; 2018. p. 136–76.

3. Algafly A, George K. The effect of cryotherapy on nerve conduction velocity, pain threshold and pain tolerance. Br J Sports Med 2007;41:365–9.

4. Feys P, Helsen W, Liu X, et al. Effects of peripheral cooling on intention tremor in multiple sclerosis. J Neurol Neurosurg Psychiatry 2005;76:373–9.

5. Secrist ES, Freedman KB, Ciccotti MG, et al. Pain management after outpatient anterior cruciate ligament reconstruction. A systematic review of randomized controlled trials. Am J Sports Med 2016;44(9):2435–47.

6. Kuyucu E, Bülbül M, Kara A, et al. Is cold therapy really efficient after knee arthroplasty? Ann Med Surg (Lond) 2015;4:475–8.

7. Quinlan P, Davis J, Fields K, et al. Effects of localized cold therapy on pain in postoperative spinal fusion patients. Orthop Nurs 2017;36:344–9.

8. Keskin C, Özdemir O, Uzun İ, et al. Effect of intracanal cryotherapy on pain after single-visit root canal treatment. Aust Endod J 2007;43:83–8.

9. Thijs E, Schotanus MG, Bemelmans YF, et al. Reduced opiate use after total knee arthroplasty using computer assisted cryotherapy. Knee Surg Sports Traumatol Arthrosc 2019;27(4):1204–12.

10. Harris J, Dhupa S. Cryotherapy. Compendium 2007;29(10):632–5.

11. Zemke JE, Andersen JC, Guion WK, et al. Intramuscular temperature responses in the human leg to two forms of cryotherapy: ice massage and ice bag. J Orthop Sports Phys Ther 1998;27(4):301–7.

12. Song M, Sun X, Tian X, et al. Compressive cryotherapy versus cryotherapy alone in patients undergoing knee surgery: a meta-analysis. Springerplus 2016;5:1074.

13. Rexing J, Dunning D, Siegel AM, et al. Effects of cold compression, bandaging, and microcurrent electrical therapy after cranial cruciate ligament repair in dogs. Vet Surg 2010;39:54–8.

14. Drygas K, McClure S, Goring R, et al. Effect of cold compression therapy on postoperative pain, swelling, range of motion, and lameness after tibial plateau leveling osteotomy in dogs. J Am Vet Med Assoc 2011;238:1284–91.

15. Okcu G, Yercan HS. Is it possible to decrease skin temperature with ice packs under casts and bandages? Arch Orthop Trauma Surg 2006;126:668–73.

16. Weresh MJ, Bennett GL, Njus G. Analysis of cryotherapy penetration: a comparison of the plaster cast, synthetic cast, Ace® wrap dressing, and Robert-Jones dressing. Foot Ankle Int 1996;1:37–40.

17. Ibrahim T, Ong SM, Saint Clair Taylor GJ. The effects of different dressings on the skin temperature of the knee during cryotherapy. Knee 2005;12:21–3.

18. Gaynor JS, Hagberg S, Gurfein BT. Veterinary applications of pulsed electromagnetic field therapy. Res Vet Sci 2018;119:1–8.

19. Rohde C, Chiang A, Adipoju O, et al. Effects of pulsed electromagnetic fields on interleukin-1 β and postoperative pain: a double-blind, placebo-controlled, pilot study in breast reduction patients. Plast Reconstr Surg 2010;125:1620–9.

20. Strauch B, Herman C, Dabb R, et al. Evidence-based use of pulsed electromagnetic field therapy in clinical plastic surgery. Aesthet Surg J 2009;29:135–43.

21. Aaron R, Ciombor DM, Simon B. Treatment of nonunions with electric and electromagnetic fields. Clin Orthop 2004;419:21–9.

22. Rawe IM, Lowenstein A, Barcelo CR, et al. Control of postoperative pain with a wearable continuously operating pulsed radiofrequency energy device: a preliminary study. Aesthetic Plast Surg 2012;36:458–63.

23. Rohde CH, Taylor EM, Alonso A, et al. Pulsed electromagnetic fields reduce postoperative interleukin-1β, pain, and inflammation: a double blind, placebo-controlled study in TRAM flap breast reconstruction patients. Plast Reconstr Surg 2015;135:808–17.

24. Hedèn P, Pilla AA. Effects of pulsed electromagnetic fields on postoperative pain: a double-blind randomized pilot study in breast augmentation patients. Aesthetic Plast Surg 2008;32:660–6.

25. Elshiwi AM, Hamada HA, Mosaad D, et al. Effect of pulsed electromagnetic field on nonspecific low back pain patients: a randomized controlled trial. Braz J Phys Ther 2019;23(3):244–9.

26. Sorrell RG, Muhlenfeld J, Moffett J, et al. Evaluation of pulsed electromagnetic field therapy for the treatment of chronic postoperative pain following lumbar surgery: a pilot, double-blind, randomized, sham-controlled clinical trial. J Pain Res 2018;11:1209–22.

27. Jung JG, Park JH, Kim SC, et al. Effectiveness of pulsed electromagnetic field for pain caused by placement of initial orthodontic wire in female orthodontic patients: a preliminary single-blind randomized clinical trial. Am J Orthod Dentofacial Orthop 2017;152:582–91.

28. Bagnato GL, Miceli G, Marino N, et al. Pulsed electromagnetic fields in knee osteoarthritis: a double blind, placebo-controlled, randomized clinical trial. Rheumatology 2016;55:755–62.

29. Yang X, He H, Gao Q, et al. Pulsed electromagnetic field improves subchondral bone microstructure in knee osteoarthritis rats through a Wnt/β-catenin signaling-associated mechanism. Bioelectromagnetics 2018;39:89–97.

30. Strauch B, Patel MK, Navarro JA, et al. Pulsed magnetic fields accelerate cutaneous wound healing in rats. Plast Reconstr Surg 2007;120:425–30.

31. Alvarez LX, McCue J, Lam NK, et al. Effect of targeted pulsed electromagnetic field therapy on canine postoperative hemilaminectomy: a double-blind, randomized, placebo-controlled clinical trial. J Am Anim Hosp Assoc 2019;55(2):83–91.

32. Zidan N, Fenn J, Griffith E, et al. The effect of electromagnetic fields on postoperative pain and locomotor recovery in dogs with acute, severe thoracolumbar intervertebral disc extrusion: a randomized placebo-controlled, prospective clinical trial. J Neurotrauma 2018;35:1726–36.

33. Shafford HL, Hellyer PW, Crump KT, et al. Use of pulsed electromagnetic field for treatment of post-operative pain in dogs: a pilot study. Vet Anaesth Analg 2002; 29:43–8.

34. Sullivan MO, Gordon-Evans WJ, Knap KE, et al. Randomized, controlled clinical trial evaluating the efficacy of pulsed signal therapy in dogs with osteoarthritis. Vet Surg 2013;42:250–4.

35. Assisi Animal Health. Available at: https://assisianimalhealth.com/vets/. Accessed June 04, 2019.

36. Johnson M, Martinson M. Efficacy of electrical nerve stimulation for chronic musculoskeletal pain: a meta-analysis of randomized controlled trials. Pain 2007;130:157–65.

37. Melzack R, Wall PD. Pain mechanisms: a new theory. Science 1965;150:971–8.

38. Sabino GS, Santos CM, Francischi JN, et al. Release of endogenous opioids following transcutaneous electric nerve stimulation in and experimental model of acute inflammatory pain. J Pain 2008;9:157–63.

39. Kalra A, Urban MO, Sluka KA. Blockade of opioid receptors in rostral ventral medulla prevents antihyperalgesia produced by transcutaneous electrical nerve stimulation (TENS). J Pharmacol Exp Ther 2001;298:257–63.

40. Sluka KA, Deacon M, Stibal A, et al. Spinal blockade of opioid receptors prevents the analgesia produced by TENS in arthritic rats. J Pharmacol Exp Ther 1999; 289(2):840–6.
41. Platon B, Mannheimer C, Andréll. Effects of high-frequency, high-intensity transcutaneous electrical nerve stimulation versus intravenous opioids for pain relief after gynecologic laparoscopic surgery: a randomized controlled study. Korean J Anesthesiol 2018;2:149–56.
42. Yilmaz E, Karakaya E, Baydur H, et al. Effect of transcutaneous electrical nerve stimulation on postoperative pain and patient satisfaction. Pain Manag Nurs 2019;20(2):140–5.
43. Kerai S, Saxena KN, Taneja B, et al. Role of transcutaneous electrical nerve stimulation in post-operative analgesia. Indian J Anaesth 2014;4:388–93.
44. Wang B, Tang J, White PF, et al. Effect of the intensity of transcutaneous acupoint stimulation on the postoperative analgesic requirement. Anesth Analg 1997;85: 406–13.
45. Bjordal JM, Johnson MI, Ljunggreen AE. Transcutaneous electrical nerve stimulation (TENS) can reduce postoperative analgesic consumption. A meta-analysis with assessment of optimal treatment parameters for postoperative pain. Eur J Pain 2003;7:181–8.
46. Li J, Song Y. Transcutaneous electrical nerve stimulation for postoperative pain control after total knee arthroplasty: a meta-analysis of randomized controlled trials. Medicine 2017;96:37.
47. Mahure SA, Rokito AS, Kwon YW. Transcutaneous electrical nerve stimulation for postoperative pain relief after arthroscopic rotator cuff repair: a prospective double-blinded randomized trial. J Shoulder Elbow Surg 2017;26:1508–13.
48. Lan F, Ma YH, Xue JX. Transcutaneous electrical nerve stimulation on acupoints reduces fentanyl requirement for postoperative pain relief after total hip arthroplasty in elderly patients. Minerva Anestesiol 2012;78:887–95.
49. Grover CA, McKernan MP, Close RJ. Transcutaneous electrical nerve stimulation (TENS) in the emergency department for pain relief: a preliminary study of feasibility and efficacy. West J Emerg Med 2018;19:872–6.
50. DeSantana JM, Walsh DM, Vance C, et al. Effectiveness of transcutaneous electrical stimulation for treatment of hyperalgesia and pain. Curr Rheumatol Rep 2008;10:492–9.
51. Levine D, Bockstahler B. Electrical stimulation. In: Millis DL, Levine D, editors. Canine rehabilitation and physical therapy. 2nd edition. Philadelphia: Saunders; 2014. p. 342–58.
52. Hanks J, Levine D, Bockstahler B. Physical agent modalities in physical therapy and rehabilitation of small animals. Vet Clin North Am Small Anim Pract 2015;45: 29–44.
53. Pryor B, Millis DL. Therapeutic laser in veterinary medicine. Vet Clin North Am Small Anim Pract 2015;45:45–56.
54. Smith JJ. General principles of laser therapy. In: Riegel RJ, Godbold JC, editors. Laser therapy in veterinary medicine. 1st edition. Chichester, West Sussex: Wiley; 2017. p. 55–66.
55. Buijs S, Godbold JC. Intra- and postoperative laser therapy. In: Riegel RJ, Godbold JC, editors. Laser therapy in veterinary medicine. 1st edition. Chichester, West Sussex: Wiley; 2017. p. 88–99.
56. Robinson NG. Photomedicine, not opioids, for chronic pain. Photomed Laser Surg 2016;34:433–44.

57. Pereira FC, Parisi JR, Maglioni CB, et al. Antinociceptive effects of low-level laser therapy at 3 and 8J/cm^2 in a rat model of postoperative pain: possible role of endogenous opioids. Lasers Surg Med 2017;49:844–51.

58. Pozzo DH, Fregapani PW, Weber JB, et al. Analgesic action of laser therapy (LLLT) in an animal model. Med Oral Patol Oral Cir Bucal 2008;13:648–52.

59. Sakurai Y, Yamaguchi M, Abiko Y. Inhibitory effect of low-level laser irradiation on LPS-stimulated prostaglandin E$_2$ production and cyclooxygenase-2 in human gingival fibroblasts. Eur J Oral Sci 2000;108:29–34.

60. White PF, Lazo OL, Galeas L, et al. Use of electroanalgesia and laser therapies as alternatives to opioids for acute and chronic pain management. F1000Res 2017; 6:2116.

61. Bjordal JM, Lopes-Martins RA, Iversen VV. A randomized, placebo controlled trial of low level laser therapy for activated Achilles tendinitis with microdialysis measurement of peritendinous prostaglandin E$_2$ concentrations. Br J Sports Med 2006;40:76–80.

62. Honmura A, Ishii A, Yanase M, et al. Analgesic effect of Ga-Al-As diode laser irradiation on hyperalgesia in carrageenan-induced inflammation. Lasers Surg Med 1993;13:463–9.

63. Ojea AR, Madi O, Neto RM, et al. Beneficial effects of applying low-level laser to surgical wounds after bariatric surgery. Photomed Laser Surg 2016;34:580–4.

64. Pereira da Silva J, Alves da Silva M, Almeida AP, et al. Laser therapy in the tissue repair process a literature review. Photomed Laser Surg 2010;28:17–21.

65. Peplow PV, Chung TY, Baxter GD. Laser photobiomodulation of wound healing: a review of experimental studies in mouse and rat animal models. Photomed Laser Surg 2010;28:291–325.

66. Meirelles GC, Santos JN, Chagas PO, et al. A comparative study of the effects of laser photobiomodulation on the healing of third-degree burns: a histological study in rats. Photomed Laser Surg 2008;26:159–66.

67. Meireles GC, Santos JN, Chagas PO, et al. Effectiveness of laser photobiomodulation at 660 or 780 nanometers on the repair of third-degree burns in diabetic rats. Photomed Laser Surg 2008;26:47–54.

68. Gonçalves WL, Souza FM, Conti CL, et al. Influence of He-Ne laser therapy on the dynamics of wound healing in mice treated with anti-inflammatory drugs. Braz J Med Biol Res 2007;40:877–84.

69. Reddy GK, Stehno-Bittel L, Enwemeka CS. Laser photostimulation accelerates wound healing in diabetic rats. Wound Repair Regen 2001;9:248–55.

70. Hawkins D, Abrahamse H. Effect of multiple exposures of low-level laser therapy on the cellular responses of wounded human skin fibroblasts. Photomed Laser Surg 2006;24:705–14.

71. Fung DT, Ng GY, Leung MC, et al. Therapeutic low energy laser improves the mechanical strength of repairing medial collateral ligament. Lasers Surg Med 2001; 31:91–6.

72. Hagiwara S, Iwasaka H, Okuda K, et al. GaAlAs (830 nm) low-level laser enhances endogenous opioid analgesia in rats. Lasers Surg Med 2007;39:797–802.

73. Ojaghi R, Sohanaki H, Ghasemi T, et al. Role of low-intensity laser therapy on naloxone-precipitated morphine withdrawal signs in mice: is nitric oxide a possible candidate mediator? Lasers Med Sci 2014;29:1655–9.

74. Nesioonpour S, Mokmeli S, Vojdani S, et al. The effect of low-level laser on postoperative pain after tibial fracture surgery: a double-blind controlled randomized clinical trial. Anesth Pain Med 2014;4:e17350.

75. Draper WE, Schubert TA, Clemmons RM, et al. Low-level laser therapy reduces time to ambulation in dogs after hemilaminectomy: a preliminary study. J Small Anim Pract 2012;53:465–9.
76. Looney AL, Huntingford JL, Blaeser LL, et al. A randomized blind placebo-controlled trial investigating the effects of photobiomodulation therapy (PBMT) on canine elbow osteoarthritis. Can Vet J 2018;59(9):959–66.
77. Marques VI, Cassu RN, Nascimento FF, et al. Laser acupuncture for postoperative pain management in cats. Evid Based Complement Alternat Med 2015; 2015:653270.
78. Kennedy KC, Martinez SA, Martinez SE, et al. Effects of low-level laser therapy on bone healing and signs of pain in dogs following tibial plateau leveling osteotomy. Am J Vet Res 2018;79:893–904.

UNITED STATES POSTAL SERVICE®
Statement of Ownership, Management, and Circulation
(All Periodicals Publications Except Requester Publications)

1. Publication Title	2. Publication Number	3. Filing Date
VETERINARY CLINICS OF NORTH AMERICA: SMALL ANIMAL PRACTICE	003 – 150	9/18/2019

4. Issue Frequency	5. Number of Issues Published Annually	6. Annual Subscription Price
JAN, MAR, MAY, JUL, SEP, NOV	6	$338.00

7. Complete Mailing Address of Known Office of Publication *(Not printer)* *(Street, city, county, state, and ZIP+4®)*

ELSEVIER INC.
230 Park Avenue, Suite 800
New York, NY 10169

Contact Person
STEPHEN R. BUSHING
Telephone *(Include area code)*
215-239-3688

8. Complete Mailing Address of Headquarters or General Business Office of Publisher *(Not printer)*

ELSEVIER INC.
230 Park Avenue, Suite 800
New York, NY 10169

9. Full Names and Complete Mailing Addresses of Publisher, Editor, and Managing Editor *(Do not leave blank)*

Publisher *(Name and complete mailing address)*

TAYLOR BALL, ELSEVIER INC.
1600 JOHN F KENNEDY BLVD. SUITE 1800
PHILADELPHIA, PA 19103-2899

Editor *(Name and complete mailing address)*

Colleen Dietzler, ELSEVIER INC.
1600 JOHN F KENNEDY BLVD. SUITE 1800
PHILADELPHIA, PA 19103-2899

Managing Editor *(Name and complete mailing address)*

PATRICK MANLEY, ELSEVIER INC.
1600 JOHN F KENNEDY BLVD. SUITE 1800
PHILADELPHIA, PA 19103-2899

10. Owner *(Do not leave blank. If the publication is owned by a corporation, give the name and address of the corporation immediately followed by the names and addresses of all stockholders owning or holding 1 percent or more of the total amount of stock. If not owned by a corporation, give the names and addresses of the individual owners. If owned by a partnership or other unincorporated firm, give its name and address as well as those of each individual owner. If the publication is published by a nonprofit organization, give its name and address.)*

Full Name	Complete Mailing Address
WHOLLY OWNED SUBSIDIARY OF REED/ELSEVIER, US HOLDINGS	1600 JOHN F KENNEDY BLVD. SUITE 1800 PHILADELPHIA, PA 19103-2899

11. Known Bondholders, Mortgagees, and Other Security Holders Owning or Holding 1 Percent or More of Total Amount of Bonds, Mortgages, or Other Securities. If none, check box ► ☐ None

Full Name	Complete Mailing Address
N/A	

12. Tax Status *(For completion by nonprofit organizations authorized to mail at nonprofit rates)* *(Check one)*
The purpose, function, and nonprofit status of this organization and the exempt status for federal income tax purposes:
☒ Has Not Changed During Preceding 12 Months
☐ Has Changed During Preceding 12 Months *(Publisher must submit explanation of change with this statement)*

PS Form **3526**, July 2014 *(Page 1 of 4 (see instructions page 4))* PSN: 7530-01-000-9931 PRIVACY NOTICE: See our privacy policy on www.usps.com.

---

13. Publication Title		14. Issue Date for Circulation Data Below
VETERINARY CLINICS OF NORTH AMERICA: SMALL ANIMAL PRACTICE		JULY 2019

15. Extent and Nature of Circulation			Average No. Copies Each Issue During Preceding 12 Months	No. Copies of Single Issue Published Nearest to Filing Date
a. Total Number of Copies *(Net press run)*			507	571
b. Paid Circulation (By Mail and Outside the Mail)	(1)	Mailed Outside-County Paid Subscriptions Stated on PS Form 3541 (Include paid distribution above nominal rate, advertiser's proof copies, and exchange copies)	311	363
	(2)	Mailed In-County Paid Subscriptions Stated on PS Form 3541 (Include paid distribution above nominal rate, advertiser's proof copies, and exchange copies)	0	0
	(3)	Paid Distribution Outside the Mails Including Sales Through Dealers and Carriers, Street Vendors, Counter Sales, and Other Paid Distribution Outside USPS®	123	147
	(4)	Paid Distribution by Other Classes of Mail Through the USPS (e.g., First-Class Mail®)	0	0
c. Total Paid Distribution *(Sum of 15b (1), (2), (3), and (4))*	►		434	510
d. Free or Nominal Rate Distribution (By Mail and Outside the Mail)	(1)	Free or Nominal Rate Outside-County Copies Included on PS Form 3541	59	42
	(2)	Free or Nominal Rate In-County Copies Included on PS Form 3541	0	0
	(3)	Free or Nominal Rate Copies Mailed at Other Classes Through the USPS (e.g., First-Class Mail)	0	0
	(4)	Free or Nominal Rate Distribution Outside the Mail (Carriers or other means)	59	42
e. Total Free or Nominal Rate Distribution *(Sum of 15d (1), (2), (3) and (4))*	►		59	42
f. Total Distribution *(Sum of 15c and 15e)*	►		493	552
g. Copies not Distributed *(See Instructions to Publishers #4 (page #3))*	►		14	19
h. Total *(Sum of 15f and g)*	►		507	571
i. Percent Paid *(15c divided by 15f times 100)*	►		88.03%	92.39%

* If you are claiming electronic copies, go to line 16 on page 3. If you are not claiming electronic copies, skip to line 17 on page 3.

16. Electronic Copy Circulation	Average No. Copies Each Issue During Preceding 12 Months	No. Copies of Single Issue Published Nearest to Filing Date
a. Paid Electronic Copies	►	
b. Total Paid Print Copies (Line 15c) + Paid Electronic Copies (Line 16a)	►	
c. Total Print Distribution (Line 15f) + Paid Electronic Copies (Line 16a)	►	
d. Percent Paid (Both Print & Electronic Copies) (16b divided by 16c × 100)	►	

☒ I certify that 50% of all my distributed copies (electronic and print) are paid above a nominal price.

17. Publication of Statement of Ownership
☒ If the publication is a general publication, publication of this statement is required. Will be printed in the NOVEMBER 2019 issue of this publication.
☐ Publication not required.

18. Signature and Title of Editor, Publisher, Business Manager, or Owner

STEPHEN R. BUSHING - INVENTORY DISTRIBUTION CONTROL MANAGER

Date 9/18/2019

I certify that all information furnished on this form is true and complete. I understand that anyone who furnishes false or misleading information on this form or who omits material or information requested on the form may be subject to criminal sanctions (including fines and imprisonment) and/or civil sanctions (including civil penalties).

PS Form **3526**, July 2014 *(Page 3 of 4)* PRIVACY NOTICE: See our privacy policy on www.usps.com

Moving?

Make sure your subscription moves with you!

To notify us of your new address, find your **Clinics Account Number** (located on your mailing label above your name), and contact customer service at:

Email: journalscustomerservice-usa@elsevier.com

800-654-2452 (subscribers in the U.S. & Canada)
314-447-8871 (subscribers outside of the U.S. & Canada)

Fax number: 314-447-8029

Elsevier Health Sciences Division
Subscription Customer Service
3251 Riverport Lane
Maryland Heights, MO 63043

*To ensure uninterrupted delivery of your subscription, please notify us at least 4 weeks in advance of move.

Printed and bound by CPI Group (UK) Ltd, Croydon, CR0 4YY

03/10/2024

01040388-0018